DISCOVERING

GOD'S
GRACE
IN
Cancer

DISCOVERING

GOD'S GRACE

IN

Cancer

A Personal Journey
with Pancreatic Cancer

Michael Seah

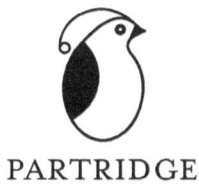

PARTRIDGE

To order additional copies of this book, contact
Toll Free 800 101 2657 (Singapore)
Toll Free 1 800 81 7340 (Malaysia)
orders.singapore@partridgepublishing.com

www.partridgepublishing.com/singapore

ACKNOWLEDGEMENTS & APPRECIATION

I am grateful to many who came alongside to provide me their love, care, encouragement and support. To each and every one of you I express my gratitude and appreciation for your faithful prayers, assistance, visitations and kind thoughts. Thank you from the bottom of my heart:

The Medical team and staff of:
Ng Teng Fong General Hospital, Singapore
Singapore Cancer Society

My immediate family:
My wife, son, daughter-in-law and grandson
My sisters and her prayerful friends
My aunts and uncles, cousins and nephews
The Millers from USA

The pastors, leaders and members of:
Adam Road Presbyterian Church
Providence Reformed Presbyterian Church
The Helping Hand

Leaders and brothers from:
Bible Study Fellowship, Singapore City Men's Evening Class

And:
All my friends and colleagues, both in Singapore and abroad who faithfully kept me in their thoughts and prayers.

A SPECIAL APPRECIATION

To my brother-in-Christ CH Chang for so patiently and diligently
reading though all my drafts and editing them so that mistakes
are corrected and points are clarified. Your suggestions are very
much appreciated. You have been an invaluable source of help.
And to all who encouraged me to share my
journey as a testimony to glorify God.
You have all made this book possible.
Thank you.

We Love to Hear From You.
Do send us your feedback and enquiries if any to:
graceincancer@yahoo.com

DEDICATION

This book is dedicated to
All who have completed, or are undergoing treatment for cancer.
And to all caregivers. whose
love and kindness is an integral part of healing.

The Lord bless you
and keep you;
the Lord make his face shine on you
and be gracious to you;
the Lord turn his face toward you
and give you peace.
Numbers 6:24-26

CONTENTS

PREFACE

As he went along, he saw a man blind from birth.
His disciples asked him, "Rabbi, who sinned, this
man or his parents, that he was born blind?"
"Neither this man nor his parents sinned," said Jesus, "but this
happened so that the works of God might be displayed in him."
John 9:1-3

Being told of having cancer must rank as one of the most difficult moments in one's life. As cancer creeps up silently, learning of its presence for the first time is very much a life changing moment. There would be a flood of emotions and concerns.

Emotions and reactions can range from fears and anxieties to quiet acceptance. There are all sorts of questions raised, ranging from its causes to treatment outcomes. Answers to these questions are not easy. There are usually few clear options and much uncertainty.

Breaking the news to family and close friends is also fraught with emotions as each one seeks to provide crucial comfort, care and support. The more religious ones would pray.

The news of my cancer came to me in a circuitous way over a couple of days of conversations and probing with the doctors. They have been trained to be cautious and not punch their patients in the face with the grim revelation. Theirs is a measured tone, explaining the prevailing medical conditions, their possible causes followed by prognosis and treatment options. The doctors' advice would be key to decisions to be made. Whatever those decisions, the treatment process is likely to be long, painful and challenging. It is important for family and friends to be alongside to provide emotional support. Their presence demonstrates love, care and concern.

For the religiously inclined, prayers help to anchor one's hopes in a sovereign God and belief in the divine power for healing.

For those who do not subscribe to a faith the spiritual aspects of healing generally may not matter. Matters of the soul and questions of life and death are very likely philosophical issues with no definitive answers. Nonetheless, many may still ponder over thoughts of death with some fear and trepidation. Whatever our individual beliefs, hopes for healing and a better day ahead are common to all.

What then is the purpose of being healed? It is obviously to prolong life so that one can live whatever remains of it to the fullest in the company of family and friends. There may still be things yet to be done, dreams to be fulfilled and hopes to be nurtured.

As a Christian, there is an added dimension of my relationship with a divine God. Only in God is there peace, solace and hope to address the deep considerations of the soul.

I found spiritual comfort in my relationship with God. I am at peace with myself under the difficult and challenging circumstances. I entrust my treatment and outcomes to the Lord because I relate to him as my Creator and Heavenly Father. My hopes for the future rest on Him and I look forward with confidence that all will be well. It is by His grace that I am assured of my future. Whatever the reasons for my illness and its consequences, a testimony of God's presence is worthy to be shared.

This then is my story of a faith journey with pancreatic cancer. Reflecting over the past months I cannot but thank God for little acts and incidents that miraculously occurred. They are more than just coincidences. They reflect how He worked in my life and was in control of my circumstances. These experiences are integral parts of my healing process. I experienced His presence and grace first-hand. His favour was upon me. I have come to appreciate Him more for His love and care.

Though some cancers today are no longer death sentences with early diagnosis, they nonetheless remain a major cause of death and many going through treatment seldom escape their fatal embrace. Knowing God brought me peace and hope in the fight against the deadly disease. His grace bestowed upon me the unmerited gift of life.

The accounts in this book are focused on God and His grace working in the course of my encounter with cancer. My narrative is only a supporting act to illustrate His presence as events unfold. This book is written with the hope of encouraging each of us to see beyond our own afflictions and to appreciate that there is a divine God who loves us.

For those who do not share my Christian beliefs, I hope you can still discover God's grace and love through events in your lives. There may be times we do not understand why things happen the way they do, yet it is possible for us to discover that there is a bright side to look forward to, and perhaps to better understand why they occurred. This is not a matter of my trying to be an optimist. God does pour His grace on everyone and we need only to acknowledge and appreciate it. We are all recipients of sunny days and rainy days. We all enjoy the beauty of His creations – the flowers, the birds, the air we breathe and the medical wisdom of doctors looking after us.

In writing this book, I will relate the events that occurred from the discovery of my cancer through its treatment process. I share my experience from a personal perspective. Interspersed between are anecdotes and reflections that have special significance for me.

Accompanying each aspect of my journey is an essay of a relevant Biblical doctrine. These doctrines reflect my understanding of the Christian faith and serve to clarify the basis of my beliefs in the context of my illness. They are not meant to be comprehensive or great in-depth studies of the topics. My understanding is gleaned from personal on-going Bible study, discussions with fellow Christians, sermons and books by reliable and established scholars. I humbly confess that I am not a Biblical scholar.

For those who have not yet embraced the Christian faith, I hope these explanations encourage you to give some serious thought to what it means to have a relationship with Jesus.

My desire is for this book to serve as a source of comfort and encouragement to those who like me, are undergoing treatment or recovering from cancer. To all caregivers, I hope it helps you to better understand and empathise with those under your care.

God is real to me and I know He wants us simply to have a closer, more intimate relationship with Him. We can all place our hopes in Him for He is our source of peace.

Finally, there is need for a small administrative clarification concerning the identities of a number of key people involved. I am identifying the doctors and other professional staff members involved in my treatment only by initials and not by name to protect their privacy and professional integrity. I have not sought permission to identify them and do not think that revealing their names is necessary. I will always be very grateful for their professionalism, high standards of care and attention. Similarly my friends in this story are also known only by their first names. If for any reason I have offended anyone by taking this approach, I humbly apologise and assume full responsibility for any errors and omissions that occurred.

Michael S Seah

March 2018

1
THE PHYSICAL, EMOTIONAL AND SPIRITUAL

Though one may be overpowered, two can defend themselves.
A cord of three strands is not quickly broken.
Ecclesiastes 4:12

A young doctor pulled a chair to my bedside and introduced himself as Dr D. He was a member of the team assigned to look after me and needed to explain the nature of my affliction. I had been admitted to the Ng Teng Fong General Hospital (NTFGH) in Singapore with acute jaundice. The results of a CT (Computed Tomography) scan done the day before are now available.

In Dr D's soft-spoken way he drew a picture of the anatomy around my stomach, pancreas and the beginning portion of my digestive system. He described how the scans have identified two lesions at the confluence of these organs. One was blocking my bile duct causing the jaundice, and the other was attached to my pancreas. He did not comment on the condition of the lesions and simply said that further investigations are needed. I probed if these lesions were actually growths and if they were malignant. He answered cautiously that they were likely to be so, subject to confirmation. He was hoping that I would not be too alarmed while preparing me for the final diagnosis to be revealed. To relieve the blockage of the bile duct a stent would have to be inserted to allow the fluids to flow. Once this was done, my jaundice should clear and the next course of action would be to deal with the lesions.

The whole process of breaking the news regarding my condition was measured and meant to be reassuring. The term "cancer" did not at any time surface in our conversations. Meanwhile a full body CT scan was ordered to see if there were other complications elsewhere in my body.

This then was my introduction to the intensive treatment undertaken by the team of medical professionals – doctors, nurses, physiotherapists, nutritionists and others at the hospital. Their sole objective was my physical recovery from the disease and how best I should be treated and cured.

The Physical, Emotional and Spiritual

News of my admission to hospital soon got to my Bible Study Fellowship (BSF) class. From the first day of admission they visited me to pray and encourage me, reassuring me of God's abiding presence. My wife, my son and his family and my sisters were also constantly by my side during visiting hours. Everyone brought me comfort and demonstrated their love and concern. Theirs was the emotional support so essential to assure me that I was not alone in my journey.

There was no doubt in my mind that my lesions were likely malignant and therefore cancerous. I was however unusually calm and not particularly anxious. I had been praying for the Lord's wisdom to guide the medical team. My family and fellow BSF leaders prayed for the Lord to be in control of all procedures and circumstances. These prayers consoled me that I had nothing to fear and I can place my trust in an almighty and loving God.

This is a spiritual realm that is dependant entirely on my faith, and my belief in a God who is all knowing and who directs all that needs to be done. He is the one who will answer our prayers. I experienced a certain calm and peace.

Over the course of the first two days or so, a patient across from my bed was observing my visitors and how each came and prayed with me. He was a friendly guy and seemed open to a conversation.

We acknowledged each other and started to talk. He asked if we are Christians and my wife and I acknowledged that we are. He introduced himself as J and though not of the same faith said he was open to the presence of a Christian God. He observed that our visitors' prayers brought me a sense of peace and confidence.

J had a bone condition in his right toe and risked having it amputated. He was anxious and worried about his future mobility. When we offered to pray for him, J had no objections and appeared comfortable and at ease. A few days later when J was told that there was no need for his toe to be amputated, he was overjoyed and thanked us for our prayers.

Fears and anxieties are common and often silently overhang over patients undergoing treatment. Comfort and peace comes only through a belief that a greater divine being is interested in our situation; cares about us; and can intervene to help us. J's condition and mine are similar in that we came to seek assurance through our belief in the power and works of God. We looked not just for physical healing and emotional support but also spiritual healing that brings peace and comfort to our souls.

Spiritual healing has to do with our deeper inner personal peace and reconciliation with a divine God. To be at peace with oneself and with God is to remove the fears and anxieties that are in us. Such peace enhances our emotional healing and helps our physical healing as well. As the title of a famous hymn goes, *It is well with my soul*.[1]

The Healing Triangle

Medical science addresses healing of the physical body. It deals with the treatment of symptoms, diagnosis of a medical condition and the procedures needed to effect a cure.

Family and friends take care of our emotional needs for daily living. They provide love and care, companionship and encouragement. This boosts our morale in challenging moments and helps lift the spirits that helps the healing process. Without emotional support we could be lonely and depression and despondency are common consequences.

The Christian faith places great importance in the concept of a family. Jesus Christ is head of the family and each believer has a part to play in support of one another.

The family in the Christian context is an extended family when we accept Jesus Christ as Lord and Saviour. The Apostle John tells us *"to those who believed in his name, he gave the right to become children of God."* (John 1:12). We are adopted into God's family and are part of the body of Christ as represented by the church and fellow believers. The author of the New Testament book of Hebrews wrote *"Both the one who makes people holy and those who are made holy are of the same family. So Jesus is not ashamed to call them brothers and sisters."* (Hebrews 2:11).

The basis for the Christian family is the love of Jesus Christ, *"A new command I give you: Love one another. As I have loved you, so you must love one another."* (John 13:34). The Apostle Paul exalted believers to *"Therefore encourage one another and build each other up"* (1 Thessalonians 5:11). The elements of emotional support are therefore integral parts of faith and spiritual support.

While physical and emotional healing takes care of the body and mind, there is the need to address matters of the heart and the soul. These deal with the deeper recesses of our emotions and include reconciling past hurts, settling grievances, and other emotions of a spiritual nature. In critical illnesses where the possibilities of death loom, there is often the need to cling to hope, to seek divine powers for healing and to be at peace in closure. These are very much matters of faith and one's beliefs.

The role of spiritual healing was drawn out in a Time magazine cover story of June 24, 1996. Among the observations highlighted, "A 1995 study at Dartmouth-Hitchcock Medical Center found that one of the best predictors of survival among 232 heart-surgery patients was the degree to which the patients said they drew comfort and strength from religious faith. Those who did not had more than three times the death rate of those who did."[2]

Religious faith appears therefore to play a significant part in the healing process. Yes, there are possible miracles in healing, those that medical science may not be able to explain. These could be in response to faithful prayers.

As Christians we believe that God our Creator, is the source of healing and peace. Jesus came as God's only Son to save us from our sins and to restore our relationship with God. There are those who do not enjoy that inner personal peace because of guilt or bitterness over things done or events in our lives. We are all born with a sinful nature and there is need for forgiveness.

In almost all religions and belief systems there is concern for this inner personal peace that resonates from the heart. In the event of death and the end of life on earth, the fears and concerns are for what happens next.

That there is life beyond our physical death is a common universal belief. This is why funeral rites are so important regardless of religious beliefs. The Egyptians mummified their pharaohs and entombed them in majestic pyramids. Many cultures bury their loved ones with all the accoutrements for a new life after death. Elaborate prayers are said to send off the dead in the hope that all would be well. Some believe in reincarnation, dependent upon the good deeds done in their lifetime. But "good" is subjective and difficult to measure. Thankfully Paul assures us *"For it is by grace you have been saved, through faith — and this is not from yourselves, it is the gift of God — not by works, so that no one can boast."* (Ephesians 2:8-9).

There are many anecdotal accounts and stories of the sick seeking healing through faith especially when all else fail. Some ignore medical science as a first source of attention in favour of faith healers. Faith alone for some may seem desirable and adequate but more often than not it does not negate the need for medical attention. God does use medical science to perform His miracles. He is after all the source of all wisdom and imparts the necessary skills to doctors.

In the midst of the healing process, we deal with our hopes and aspirations, our fears and anxieties, and our relationships with those around us. There could possibly be conflicts, confusion and uncertainties.

Healing is therefore seemingly incomplete when only the physical and emotional elements are applied. For healing to be holistic, spiritual healing must take place as well. Together they become the "cord of three strands" that is not easily broken.

Our physical, emotional and spiritual dimensions form a triangle (Figure 1) with God at its apex. From Him flows knowledge and wisdom that guide medical sciences. The link between our emotional and spiritual healing is dependant on our beliefs. Can we trust God with our needs? What if I should die?

Answers to such questions go beyond our logical and human wisdom. They can only come from our belief in a God with whom we can relate to and on whom we can anchor our hopes and prayers.

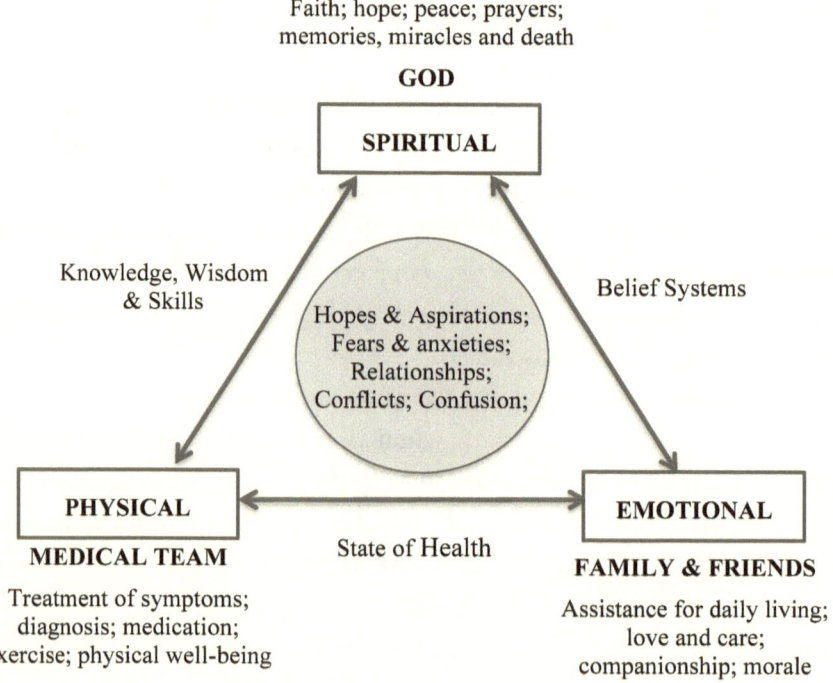

Figure 1: The Healing Triangle

God's Presence in Anxieties

Some anxieties in the course of treatment cannot be easily allayed on their own. Calming my anxieties meant turning to God in prayer and seeking His presence. For me, God's presence came through the Holy Spirit and His Word. Paul assures us: *"Do not be anxious about anything, but in every situation, by prayer and petition, with thanksgiving, present your requests to God. And the peace of God, which transcends all understanding, will guard your hearts and your minds in Christ Jesus."* (Philippians 4:6-7).

Under such circumstances, I go to God in faith. In him I place my hopes for healing, peace and perhaps some miracles. Indeed medical miracles are happening everyday around the world regardless of one's beliefs. This is God's universal grace at work. Spiritual comfort however comes only through that special relationship with Him. It is secured by acknowledging Him as the only God in our lives. God's abundant grace is unconditional when His children in Christ, go to Him.

*****

A Unique Godly Relationship

Central to the Christian faith is the doctrine of the Trinity. An understanding of our relationship with God starts with appreciating that God is a triune God. He is God in three persons and yet one. The Westminster Confession of Faith states that: "In the unity of the Godhead there be three Persons of one substance, power, and eternity: God the Father, God the Son, and God the Holy Ghost."[3] In addressing the Israelites in the desert Moses proclaimed: *"Hear, O Israel: The Lord our God, the Lord is one."* (Deuteronomy 6:4).

God is our Heavenly Father. Jesus is his Son who came in human form to die on the cross, so that mankind through his personal sacrifice may be reconciled to God. Just like a sacrificial lamb, Jesus took our sins upon himself when he died. Three days after his crucifixion Jesus rose from the dead and reappeared to his disciples. Following His resurrection and ascension to heaven, He sent the Holy Spirit (Ghost) to dwell in us as believers. In this way, God's presence is always with those of us who accept Jesus as Lord and Saviour. His Holy Spirit in us allows for a close and intimate relationship with God the Father.

Children of God.

God created man in His image. (Genesis 1:27) As such ours is a special relationship with Him. When man sinned and rebelled against a holy God that relationship was fractured. God's plan was for our redemption from sin and to be restored to Him. The Bible is the story of this redemption plan through His Son Jesus Christ.

Believing in Jesus is our first step in the restoration process. We are adopted as children of God establishing a whole new relationship with God. John explains, *"See what great love the Father has lavished on us, that we should be called children of God!"* (1 John 3:1)

As with any relationship, its bonds depend on our effort, time and commitment. The more we nurture that relationship, the stronger will be the bonds that bind resulting in greater confidence and trust. God does not fail us even though we are more likely to fail Him.

It is therefore fitting that as His children, we can approach our Heavenly Father directly in conversation, in prayer. As we praise and worship God we honour Him for who He is. Jesus having ascended into heaven sits at the right hand of God as our High Priest interceding for us (Hebrews 4:14). We are to pray in Jesus' name *"so that the Father may be glorified in the Son."* (John 14:13).

The intimacy that Jesus has with His Father, is the same intimacy we can have with God. We need to seek Him, not just in our moments of need. He is close to us as we listen to Him and discover His will and intentions through His Word. Quiet time with Him each day accords us intimate moments with Him. When we are strapped for time in the midst of our busy day, pause for a moment's conversation. Thank Him for whatever He has done, speak to Him while on the move as we would with a friend alongside. Speak aloud, or in a soft whisper, or quietly in your heart. He hears and knows what is on our hearts and in our minds. God is omnipresent. He is everywhere and He is with every believer because the Holy Spirit is in us.

Time set aside for the Lord is precious and should be a priority in itself. It is the expression of our love for Him.

Praise, Worship and Sacraments

Christianity is about our relationship with a holy God. It is unique in that it requires no special rituals or offerings in worship apart from ourselves coming to our Heavenly Father with open hearts and living lives pleasing to Him. We praise God to remind us of His attributes and His majesty. God is worthy of our worship, honour and praise.

To be a Christian requires only a short Sinner's Prayer acknowledging our sinful nature and accepting Jesus as our Lord and Saviour. We acknowledge and seek forgiveness for our sinful ways. We invite the Holy Spirit into our lives. It is a prayer we can say quietly anywhere and anytime we are prompted to. We repeat it in the presence of a fellow believer to enable a witness to the commitment of our faith and acceptance into the family of God.

Upon accepting Jesus into our lives, the next commitment is baptism. The Shorter Catechism identifies baptism as a sacrament that "signify and seal our ingrafting into Christ, and partaking of the benefits of the covenant of grace, and our engagement to be the Lord's."[4] Sacraments are "holy signs and seals of the covenant of grace"[5] and Baptism is one which is the public declaration of our faith and formal membership into the church of Christ.

With the acceptance of Christ as our Lord, we can then partake of the sacrament of Holy Communion. Jesus shared the bread and the wine with His disciples the night before He was crucified saying that they represent His body and His blood. These elements were to be taken in remembrance of Him. Today, we celebrate the Lord's Supper as the disciples did (Matt 26:26-28) in remembrance of Jesus who died on the cross that we may have life.

God's demands on us are not onerous. We are to simply, *"Love the Lord your God with all your heart and with all your soul and with all your mind." This is the first and greatest commandment.* (Matthew 22:37-38). All that we do seeks to build on and secure that unique relationship with God, our Father in Heaven.

*****

REFERENCES

1. Spafford, H. G. (Composer). (1873). *It Is Well With My Soul.*
2. Wallis, C. (1996, June 24). *Faith and Healing.* Retrieved July 18, 2017 from Time Magazine - The Vault: http://time.com/vault/issue/1996-06-24/page/113/
3. The Westminster Confession of Faith. Chapter II, 3.
4. The Westminster Confession of Faith, The Shorter Catechism. Q. 94
5. The Westminster Confession of Faith. Chapter XXIX, 1.

2
THE SUFFICIENCY OF HIS GRACE

But he said to me, "My grace is sufficient for you, for my power is made perfect in weakness." Therefore I will boast all the more gladly about my weaknesses, so that Christ's power may rest on me.
2 Corinthians 12:9

Visiting hours were over. The lights were dimmed so that patients could rest for the night. As I lay in bed looking out of the large glass window, my mind wandered into moments of reflection. I told myself that this time in hospital would be an extended quiet time with the Lord. It should be a time of prayer and conversation with God.

Extended Quiet Time and Reflections

In my extended quiet time I intended to read my Bible, meditate on the Word and be in conversation with the Lord. The evenings in hospital however had their distractions. There were times I contemplated past events or what the future holds and challenges ahead. Sleep usually was intermittent and my quiet time became a mixture of unstructured thoughts, abbreviated prayers and disconnected conversations with God.

My thoughts were thankfully, not quite those of fear or anxiety. There were moments when I reflected on past decisions in my life and wished I could have decided differently. I pondered on lessons learnt.

All too often these pointed towards self-reliance and trusting in my own abilities and instincts.

Though I came to know the Lord in the early nineteen-sixties I had slid away many years due to family objections and a focus on work and career prospects. I was not with God during that time. I returned to Him only in the early nineties when my son wanted to be baptised. He had accepted the Lord in secondary school and through him a short while later, I too found the Lord again. In reality even though I left the Lord, He never left me.

The first few quiet nights in the ward were disrupted by a noisy patient across from my bed. Late in the evenings this elderly man would get into a loud conversation with himself, or worse, sing aloud. It was a din that went on for several nights with the rest of us hoping that he could be sedated. The nurses must have been at their wit's end and finally one evening they wheeled his bed out to an isolated area when his monologue started. There, I guess he could sing himself to sleep.

When sleep finally came for me it was interrupted by times for medication or the taking of vital signs like blood pressure and body temperatures. Each morning at five, the nurses would come round for the blood tests. These had to be done so that the results could be ready when the doctors come around for their morning visits. Getting back to sleep was often a challenge. The nurses were always apologetic but then I appreciated that they were only doing their job.

Treatment Proposed

Around mid-morning of the fifth day I was brought down for my full body CT scan. We proceeded down through corridors and lifts away from public view. Before each procedure was done, patients identify themselves and were verified against the records in the system. Procedures were necessarily strict to minimise errors and to ensure that correct tests were done.

Before my scan commenced, I had to ingest some fluids to enhance the images. It was a large volume and not exactly a comfortable experience. Having done so, I was left lying on a flat bed and moved through a tunnel of spinning technology taking the most amazing continuous pictures of my interior organs. This to me can only be invented with inspiration from a divine source. As the scan came to an end, I was wheeled back to the ward through the same private corridors. All in, the whole process took probably close to an hour.

The days in the ward showed me just how vulnerable I could be. I have been afflicted by an ailment and there was very little I could do about it. I have absolutely no idea how the two lesions got in my body. My condition was in the hands of my doctors. My options were limited and all I could do was to await the results of the tests and their recommendations for treatment. I was totally dependent on their medical knowledge and could only pray that God would grant them the requisite wisdom and guidance. I had no control over my condition nor was I able to change the course of events. Only my faith tells me that God is in control.

A day later, Dr D informed me of the results of my CT scan. He told me that they had discovered a small cyst in my thyroid gland. It needed a closer look. Apart from that there were no other indications of abnormalities elsewhere in my body. Arrangements were made for me to have a tissue sample extracted from the cyst for a biopsy. It seems a second complication was afoot.

The next morning, I was wheeled down to a specialist clinic to have the biopsy done. The process involved a fine needle probe inserted into the cyst in the thyroid gland to extract the sample. I was given a local anaesthetic to dull the pain. It was relatively quick and in no time I was back at the ward. I informed my family and friends of my new condition and we prayed for a good outcome. I was in God's hands and He would direct whatever needed to be done.

Dr D came around the ward again to speak to me about my two lesions. He was now preparing me for an endoscopy, a procedure to put a probe down my throat and into the area where the lesions were located. This was to either place a stent to allow the bile to flow or to extract a tissue sample for biopsy. The medical team were in discussions on the options and priorities. Both actions carried some risks and posed possible complications for the next phase of treatment.

The results for my thyroid biopsy came back the following day. The good news was that the cyst was benign and nothing needed to be done about it.

That evening the leader of my medical team Dr L came to visit. He had seen me over the course of the previous days but now he was there with me on his own. He smiled reassuringly and drew up beside my bed with the movable bedside table drawn close. I sat up to listen to what he had to say.

Dr L is a senior consultant surgeon at the hospital. He explained the condition concerning my bile duct and pancreas. They have decided that I needed an operation to remove the two lesions. It would be a major operation involving what is known as the Whipple procedure.

It became obvious to me that my two lesions were actually two small cancerous tumours and their early removal was essential to prevent the spread of cancer cells beyond their current locations. Chemotherapy and radiotherapy were not suitable options in my case. These tumours Dr L said, if not removed early would incur the risk of growing and changing within a short space of time. Time was therefore of the essence. Without too much of a second thought, I responded, "Let's do it."

Dr L must have been taken aback at my prompt agreement to proceed. He had explained the nature of the operation and the risks involved. This was going to be a major operation taking between six and ten hours to complete without any complications. He reassured me that he was prepared to make available all the tests results and diagnosis for me to submit for a second opinion. I replied confidently that that would not be necessary. I had full confidence in his judgement and the capabilities of the team.

I do not know what brought about my confidence to proceed with the operation as recommended. I seemed impulsive and without fear or anxiety. My quiet peace can only be attributed to the Holy Spirit within me.

Dr L informed me that the hospital's Cancer Board would review the treatment strategy. The Board comprises a body of medical experts in their respective fields of speciality and include members from the National University Hospital (NUH). It is very much an internal review and audit process. Dr L would meanwhile proceed to schedule a suitable date given that I would also need time to recover from jaundice.

Concerns and Trusting God

As my family and friends came to visit, I shared with them the proposed treatment strategies and the Whipple procedure to come. None of us had heard of the Whipple procedure. The fact that it was going to be such a major operation with considerable risks evoked some concern.

As I lay in bed that night contemplating the operation to come, my thoughts revolved around the preparations needed, and how this journey was unfolding. I prayed and sought the Lord's presence and peace.

Dr D had in one of our conversations pointed to the location of the lesion blocking my bile duct. He said that it was fortuitous that the lesion was positioned in such a way that it caused jaundice. Had it been slightly off by only a fraction of a few millimetres, I may not have had any symptoms. The jaundice was in fact an important early indicator of the malignant condition. Had there been no jaundice the lesions would have grown unnoticed until it was too late for effective treatment. It was indeed a blessing that I had the jaundice to enable the discovery of the more serious condition. I realised then that God had intervened.

Earlier in May 2016, I had my annual check-up with our family physician. The results for my blood tests indicated an elevation in the cancer markers. My doctor and I discussed its implications and decided that we should monitor it. There was a possibility of a false positive reading as sometimes experienced in the past. So as not to cause too much anxiety he suggested I return for another test in August. I left that at the back of my mind and missed my appointment for August. It was hardly a month later in mid September that my jaundice surfaced and I had to make my humble visit to his clinic again. God did not allow me to forgo that important examination.

God is truly sovereign, all knowing and in control so that I was driven to receive the medical attention I needed. One might claim that it was possibly a matter of chance and good fortune. The truth however is revealed in examining events over a course of time to appreciate that these were divine interventions. My faith tells me that God was at work.

As I mentally replayed the string of events that led me to this point I cannot help but see God's grace at work. Our family physician whom we have consulted for more than twenty years is a fellow believer. He had been very conscientious about monitoring our health. He made it a point that I have an annual screening to make sure that all is well. We are blessed in having someone who is both physician and caring friend.

My early diagnosis through jaundice allows for prompt and early intervention. I have a medical team who was thoroughly professional in their approach and duties. I was admitted to a brand new hospital that is within the neighbourhood where we live. All these were not mere coincidences. I could not on my own have arranged for these to be so neatly orchestrated. God foresaw my needs and these arrangements were only possible because of His grace working out for me.

*****

God's Grace

Dr Philip Ryken, Senior Minister of Tenth Presbyterian Church, Philadelphia wrote "Theologians make a distinction between the grace God shows his people in salvation (saving grace) and the grace he shows to humanity in general (common grace). God has not reserved all his gifts for Christians."[1]

Paul's letter to the Ephesians explains *"For it is by grace you have been saved, through faith – and this not from yourselves, it is the gift of God – not by works, so that no one can boast."* (Ephesians 2:8-9). Our salvation from a life of sin and death is an unmerited gift from God given entirely by his grace through faith.

Sola Gratia, by grace alone, is one of the key principles of the Reformation. The late James Montgomery Boice tells us that "sinners have no claim upon God, none at all; that God owes them nothing but punishment for their sins, and that, if he saves them in spite of their sins … it is only because it pleases him to do it and for no other reason."[2]

Snodgrass in his commentary clarifies "Grace means the completely underserved, loving commitment of God to us. For some reason unknown to us, but which is rooted in his nature, God gives himself to us, attaches himself to us, and acts to rescue us."[3] And so, as we express our faith in Jesus Christ as our saviour, God's saving grace is poured out to us, that we will have eternal life with him. *"For as in Adam all die, so in Christ all will be made alive."* (1 Corinthians 15:22)

Our salvation is the very purpose Jesus died on the cross. His death was the price paid so that we are redeemed from a life of sin. To be saved is to be forgiven of our sins and to have the assurance of eternal life allowing us to return to God in glory when our lives end here on earth. This is the gospel – the message of reconciliation with God and one that Christians share all over the world as the "good news". Jesus before ascending to heaven gave this great commission to his followers *"Therefore go and make disciples of all nations, baptizing them in the name of the Father and of the Son and of the Holy Spirit, and teaching them to obey everything I have commanded you."* (Matthew 28:19-20).

Common grace on the other hand, is God's universal gift to all mankind. We see His grace in His creations, the air we breathe, the sky and the planetary systems, the creatures that roam the earth, the plants we consume for food, the water we need for survival. *"He has shown kindness by giving you rain from heaven and crops in their seasons; he provides you with plenty of food and fills your hearts with joy. … Rather, he himself gives everyone life and breath and everything else."* (Acts 14:17; 17:25)

All of God's creation is not restricted only for the enjoyment of Christians but for all mankind. Today's advancements in medical sciences are all part of God's common grace. These inventions, innovations and discoveries are given to us from the wisdom of God. Common grace is God's unconditional gift to mankind. It speaks of the universality of God, a God for all peoples and all nations.

To see Him work in our lives in many unexplainable ways is to experience His grace. We live in a sinful and fallen world and there are consequences to all of our actions. Each new day that we have is by His grace.

My having cancer may be due to my personal lifestyle or circumstances beyond my knowledge or control. God's grace was there to help me recover from the episode. I am closer to Him by drawing upon Him as my Heavenly Father. I go to Him in prayer and humble repentance receiving His love and presence in return. It is His grace that brings comfort, peace and even joy in difficult circumstances.

We can give thanks to God for all the little common grace experienced everyday. A simple act of thanksgiving performed by Christians everywhere everyday is also called grace. We give thanks to the Almighty for the food we eat at each meal. It is by His grace that we have food on the table and we in turn invite Him to bless the food unto our bodies. The next time you enjoy a meal, pause and give thanks to the source of your provisions.

Our God is a gracious God as the psalmist declares:

> The Lord is gracious and compassionate, slow to anger and
> rich in love.
> The Lord is good to all he has compassion on all he has made.
> (Psalm 145:8-9)

I pray for all of us that we will not just enjoy God's common grace, but also come to know Jesus and receive His gift of saving grace.

*****

REFERENCES

1. Ryken, P. G. (2004). *He Speaks to Me Everywhere - Meditations on Christianity and Culture.* Phillipsburg, New Jersey, USA: P&R Publishing Company. p15

2. Boice, J. M. (2001). *Whatever Happened To The Gospel of Grace?* Wheaton, Illinois, USA: Crossway. p107

3. Snodgrass, K. (1996). *Ephesians - The NIV Application Commentary.* Grand Rapids, Michigan, USA: Zondervan. p103

*****

3
PREPARING FOR SURGERY

Praise the Lord, my soul; all my inmost being, praise his holy name.
Praise the Lord, my soul, and forget not all his benefits—
who forgives all your sins and heals all your diseases,
who redeems your life from the pit and crowns
you with love and compassion,
who satisfies your desires with good things so that
your youth is renewed like the eagle's.
Psalm 103:1-5

By now, I had spent almost a week in hospital. My arms and hands ached from the countless injections to draw blood for tests. These were daily occurrences and multiple times within a day. I also had a needle with a plug called a "cannula", attached to one of my hands or arms seemingly permanently for intravenous injections. These cannulas were changed every three days so that they do not become contaminated. One of my friends visiting me remarked that when he was hospitalised some time back, the blood they drew from him could have filled a swimming pool. I laughed at my own circumstance and said that I was not too far away from his experience.

Seeking a Second Opinion

The news of my undergoing a Whipple procedure aroused some cautionary response and concerns from family and friends. My son was advised to have me seek a second opinion. His friends knew how difficult and risky the operation was. Some suggested that it might be good for me to be transferred to another general hospital with greater experience in the Whipple procedure. Literature on the Whipple procedure all pointed to success being dependent on the doctors' experience and the facilities available at major hospitals. Our family physician told me to ascertain the experience of the hospital staff with the Whipple. Two other friends who met their doctor friends also expressed the same concerns when they described the complexities involved.

I took note of all these comments and expressed my confidence in the hospital and the team involved. I felt that being a new major general hospital does not mean that the medical team was new and inexperienced. I had prayed and placed my trust in the Lord to direct my medical treatment. I believed He had directed me to the place He wanted me to be.

I experienced God's peace within me and decided not to seek a second opinion or a transfer to another hospital. The latter was likely to result in delays and possibly a whole series of new tests. It would also increase inconveniences for travel and visitations. I have placed my trust in the Lord and until there were clear signs that I should change, I shall not do so.

Dealing With The Tumours

Dr D and his colleagues were now preparing me for the operation to come. The Cancer Board recommended that I should have the biopsy done on the tumour to determine its specific nature before implanting a stent to drain my blocked fluids.

In addition to determining the nature of the tumours, Dr D was concerned that all other micro cancer cells should also be discovered. These may be hidden and are not detectable by the CT scans. He strongly recommended that I undertake a PET (Positron Emission Tomography) scan to try and detect these possibilities.

A PET scan with its radioactive glucose based solution will be better at identifying possible clusters of cancer cells. I was told that cancer cells feed on glucose. Arrangements for the PET scan had to be made with an external facility. The scan will give a better assurance that the cancer had not spread. I agreed to the scan and arrangements were made for me to have an urgent appointment with the facility.

Early the next morning an ambulance arrived to take me for the PET scan. A nurse accompanied me on the journey and we arrived a little after seven. I was told to drink some two litres of a sweet concoction. Once ready, the full body scan proceeded as planned. I was told that the images would highlight clusters of glucose where cancer cells are found. The state of medical technology amazes me and I was just thankful that I was able to receive such high standards of medical care and attention.

After the scan was completed, another ambulance was called to return me to the hospital. It was almost time for lunch when we arrived back at the ward. It had been a tiring exercise.

Dr D was delighted when he met me the next day. The PET scan indicated clearly that the cancer cells had not spread. I was cleared for the operation as planned. The date set was 24 October, a Monday some three weeks away. Meanwhile I could be discharged within the next few days to return home to rest and rebuild myself.

The endoscopy to obtain a biopsy had been arranged. I was brought down to the theatre and sedated for the procedure. The whole process took the better part of an afternoon and the sedation was helpful in that I felt no discomfort while the tissue sample was being extracted.

In the midst of all these activities, my jaundice had not subsided. I was still experiencing its effects and feeling lethargic. I slept whenever I could and generally had little energy to last a whole day. My appetite was not particularly great and I was losing some weight. Dr D saw me again and opined that the stent could not be delayed.

A second endoscopy was ordered. I was once again wheeled to the theatre and sedated. The difference this time was that the sedation did not cover the full duration of the procedure due to a slight fever. I awoke somewhere towards the end of the procedure and could hear the conversations with regards to the work being done on me. I was in great discomfort throughout the remaining half hour or so. Finally, it was all over and the implements removed from my mouth. Oh, what a relief!

As Dr D came to see me the next morning, I was in much better shape. Apparently my temperature was back to normal and blood tests indicated a significant drop in my jaundice markers. The stent was working as intended. I prayed, thanking God for the good outcome.

Preparation for Discharge

The best news for me was when Dr D appeared later in the day to announce that I would remain in the hospital for another day or two for observation. If there were no adverse developments he would discharge me and allow me to return home. I had been in hospital some ten days and I was looking forward to being home.

As part of the preparation for my discharge, the physiotherapists visited me to confirm that I was physically strong and steady enough to move around on my own. We first took a walk around the vicinity of the ward just to make sure that I was sufficiently mobile. I was taken in a wheelchair up to a special gym where I demonstrated my ability to cope with climbing stairs and getting on and off public transport. The physiotherapists congratulated me on my abilities and declared that they had no reservations about my ability to move about on my own.

My visitors and family observed that I was looking much better and seemingly in good spirits. For now, all our prayers had been answered and God was truly with me through this part of the journey.

On the thirteenth day, Sunday 9 October, Dr D signed off my discharge papers in the morning and I prepared to return home. The discharge procedures included not just the financial matters but also coordination with the pharmacy for medications I required and a readmission appointment for my operation. When all was done, I changed into my normal clothes and walked out of the ward with my wife by my side. I said my good byes and thanked the nursing staff for their wonderful dedication and care. To the few familiar fellow patients we wished each other speedy recovery and God's blessings. Francis, a close friend came to drive us home.

Those thirteen eventful days taught me to trust God and draw closer to Him. It had been an experience that brought family and friends together and showed me the love and care they have for me. Above all, I know how real God is and how He was with me all this while, though unseen. I gained an inner peace and assurance that my sovereign Lord was in control and directing me through the treatment I needed.

Time at Home and With God

As I read the Psalms one morning at home, I was led to Psalm 103. I was looking for words of assurance from the Lord. His promise to heal all my diseases and restore my youth spoke to me loud and clear.

Psalm 103 spoke of so many of God's attributes wrapped in His promises. He is holy and worthy of our praise. He forgives, He heals, and He redeems us from our sinful ways. He is compassionate and His love for us fills our desires with good things. He means only good for us. He is our restorer bringing back our youth so that we are renewed. He helps us soar once again like eagles, to the high points of our lives. What more can I ask for? I can but only praise His holy name. God is good!

I could not have asked for a more specific assurance. O Lord my God, great is your faithfulness for they are new every morning! Your grace is more than sufficient for me.

Around this time, my son and his family were in the process of preparing to return to the United States. My son had been expecting his visa approval anytime soon. However, there seemed to be a unexpected delay. Given my medical condition, this delay turned out to be a blessing in disguise. Had my son and his family returned to the States in June as originally anticipated, they would have left feeling anxious and worried about my condition. It would have been difficult for them to decide about returning to Singapore to be by my side. Now that the visa had not been issued, we all found great comfort being together during these weeks of stress and uncertainty.

We would also have greatly missed our grandson being here with us. One of the best moments during the two weeks at home was when he came to visit. He is a bright bubbly boy who had just celebrated his eighth birthday in early September. He has this wonderful love for and knowledge of dinosaurs and we could spend all day listening to his tales about them. There were also wonderful moments creating imaginative conversations and stories with his collection of dinosaurs together with a mixture of Lego bricks and Disney characters. Yes, I would have sorely missed his smile, his laughter and his innocent sense of humour.

Then there was my wife's retirement earlier in the year. She decided to opt for retirement in order to spend more time with our grandson. Had she been still working, it would have been very difficult and stressful for her to be shuttling between work and hospital to attend to me. God ensured her retirement would give her time to attend to my needs.

These events showed to me that there was certainly some divine intervention in all these circumstances. God was directing these events such that I did not miss the treatment I needed while having the presence of my family by my side at the most crucial moments. He was demonstrably and undoubtedly in control. I was now home on a two-week break to prepare myself physically, emotionally and spiritually for the more challenging phase of my treatment.

*****

God's Sovereignty

The Westminster Confession states, "God from all eternity did by the most wise and holy counsel of his own will, freely and unchangeably ordain whatsoever comes to pass; yet so as thereby neither is God the author of sin, nor is violence offered to the will of the creatures, nor is the liberty or contingency of second causes taken away, but rather established."[1] This declaration underscores that God from the very beginning by His own will establishes and creates all things, allowing for all events and activities to occur. Nothing is created, or is done, or gets affected without His sovereign knowledge and will.

R. C. Sproul explains "that God neither commits sin Himself, nor does He work in such a manner that He coerces His creatures to sin. At the same time the Confession avows that God ordains whatever comes to pass. He ordains the actions of human beings but not in such a way that He does violence to the will of His creatures or nullifies second causes."[2] Sproul refers second causes to the "the force imparted by physical creatures."[3]

One discussion on God's sovereignty revolves around the expression of his supreme powers over creation, the peoples of the world and the events that shape their lives. "The meaning of the sovereignty of God is that human beings are, at every moment of our lives, in relationship to the living God."[4] It is the essence and quality of this relationship that defines God to us.

References to God's Sovereignty

In the New International Version (NIV) Bible, the patriarch Abraham and leaders of the Israel like Moses, Joshua, King David and a number of prophets all used the term "Sovereign Lord" in reference to God.

Moses proclaimed, "Sovereign Lord, you have begun to show to your servant your greatness and your strong hand. For what god is there in heaven or on earth who can do the deeds and mighty works you do?" (Deuteronomy 3:24).

King David in praise declared, *"Yours, Lord, is the greatness and the power and the glory and the majesty and the splendor, for everything in heaven and earth is yours."* (1 Chronicles 29:11).

God's Attributes

God is timeless. *"In the beginning God created the heavens and the earth."* (Genesis 1:1). He was there at the beginning even before time began. His sovereignty is derived from His character. He is omnipotent – His powers are limitless. He is omnipresent – His presence is everywhere at all times.

And, He is omniscient – He is an all-knowing God. *"I am God, and there is no other; I am God, and there is none like me."* (Isaiah 46:9).

R. C. Sproul, points to a God who had the option not to forgive us but to destroy us for our sins. Yet, in His grace and mercies He chose to provide opportunities for salvation.[5] God works to fulfill His plans.

God knows and is in Control

One question often asked concerning God's sovereignty relates to why God allows evil and disasters to befall mankind? If God is in control and He loves us, why then does He allow us to get sick with cancer, or worse perish in the midst of accidents, natural disasters, or in events of terrorism? Surely a God who is all powerful and all knowing can prevent all these from happening.

Such questions are not unreasonable. Their answers are not easy and involve the mysteries of God that we cannot fully understand. Nothing happens outside the knowledge and will of God.

God's people do not escape suffering from pain and disappointments even though we are often reminded of what Paul wrote in Romans 8:28 - *"And we know that in all things God works for the good of those who love him, who have been called according to his purpose."*

Sproul refers to the story of how Joseph's brothers, in an evil plot to get rid of him, sold him off to merchants, but God turned the plot around to save the Israelites from famine.[6] Joseph on reuniting with his brothers said to them, *"I am your brother Joseph, the one you sold into Egypt! And now, do not be distressed and do not be angry with yourselves for selling me here, because it was to save lives that God sent me ahead of you. ... You intended to harm me, but God intended it for good to accomplish what is now being done, the saving of many lives."* (Genesis 45:4-5; 50:20).

For many of us who experienced pain and suffering, understanding God's sovereign plan and will in our lives is not easy especially when there is an unexplainable and unknown period of time before God's goodness and plans become obvious.

Following the massive Indian Ocean tsunami in December 2004, Arjith Fernando, National Director for Sri Lanka Youth for Christ wrote, "Asking why a terrible thing happened is one aspect of biblical lament. ... Usually at the end of a time of grappling, God's people affirm that because God is sovereign and knows what is happening, the wisest thing is to keep trusting Him. Believing in God's sovereignty at a time of tragedy helps us to avoid hopelessness amidst the struggle. We must rely on God's promise that even out of terrible tragedy, He will bring something good to those who love Him."[7]

God's sovereignty does not infringe on man's own will. The Westminster Confession declares, "God hath endued the will of man with that natural liberty, that it is neither forced, nor by any absolute necessity of nature determined to good or evil."[8] We each have the liberty to decide and to come to our own decisions in all matters of our lives. We can choose to live a life that is pleasing to God or choose to depart from His ways.

*****

REFERENCES

1. The Westminster Confession of Faith. Chapter III, 1.
2. Sproul, R. C. (1996). *The Invisible Hand.* Phillipsburg, New Jersey, USA: P&R Publishing. p80
3. Ibid. p104
4. The United Presbyterian Church in the USA. (1999). Introduction to the Westminster Standards. In *Book of Confessions* (Study Edition ed., p. 169). Louisville, Kentucky, USA: Geneva Press.
5. Sproul, R. C. (2017). *Chosen By God - God's Sovereignty.* Retrieved july 24, 2017 from Ligonier Ministries, the teaching fellowship of R.C. Sproul: http://www.ligonier.org/learn/series/chosen_by_god/gods-sovereignty/
6. Sproul, R. C. (1996). *The Invisible Hand.* Phillipsburg, New Jersey, USA: P&R Publishing. p87-96
7. Fernando, A. (2005). *After the Tsunami.* Grand Rapids, Michigan, USA: RBC Ministries.
8. The Westminster Confession of Faith. Chapter XI, 1.

4

MY PANCREATIC CANCER AND SURGERY

Whoever dwells in the shelter of the Most High
will rest in the shadow of the Almighty.
I will say of the Lord, "He is my refuge and my fortress,
my God, in whom I trust."
Psalm 91:1-2

Trusting the Lord can sound almost like a cliché until real events overwhelm and reliance on Him is not an option. It is all too easy to advise someone to trust God when the consequences do not affect us personally. Would God come through and would prayers be answered?

Our relationship with God is personal. Like all relationships, trust depends on the bond that exists. Trust comes with confidence that one will act in the interest of the other even at a cost. Central to Christian belief is the knowledge that God's love for his people came at the very high and painful cost of his son Jesus dying on the cross as a sacrificial lamb to atone for the sins of mankind. Believing in Jesus is acknowledging that sacrifice and trusting God in a relationship where we are his beloved children. To trust God is to believe that He is a promise keeping God. He will not fail us the way our fellow men fail us and we fail others.

When we trust God we look to Him as our refuge and our fortress (Psalm 91). The psalmist exalts God for His protection and the assurance of His presence in the most difficult of circumstances.

Drawing Closer to God

As my operation drew closer, I felt a sense of peace, surrendering whatever the outcome entirely into God's hands. It was a strange feeling knowing that I had no control over the course of events.

During the two weeks at home I sought time alone with the Lord in quiet contemplation. It was in such moments that the Lord spoke to me through Psalms 103 and 91. Both psalms speak of God's promise of protection and restoration. They provide the assurance of God's presence in difficult and challenging circumstances. It was in one of these moments that I plucked up courage and said, "Lord, help me. I want to live."

Over the course of the days at home, my wife and I had conversations about tidying up my affairs and what should be done in the event that the Lord calls me home. I arranged to settle my will and drafted instructions ranging from funeral arrangements to disposing my personal possessions.

While I was quietly confident of a good outcome, I did at times wonder if all my preparations for the worst-case scenario reflected my trust or lack thereof in the Lord. We have all prayed. We have all said we put our trust in Him. We have all believed that our prayers will be answered. Yet here is Plan B in case something happens. What a apparent contradiction. It was all too easy to simply say, "Trust the Lord." I convinced myself that I was just being practical.

Thoughts on Cancer

My readings on cancer were at best cursory. I understood generally what cancer is but until now can only sympathise with those afflicted with the disease. Within my family several members died of cancer and my doctors wondered if mine was hereditary and in my DNA.

Pancreatic cancer is one of the more notorious forms of cancers. The World Cancer Report 2014, noted that it was the seventh most common cause of cancer deaths.[1] According to the Mayo Clinic's web site, pancreatic cancer typically spreads rapidly and is seldom detected in its early stages.[2]

The Whipple Procedure

My diagnosis for pancreatic cancer was deemed early enough to be operable. Dr L described the operation as one with a curative objective.

The Whipple procedure was named after Allen Whipple, an American surgeon, who did the surgery in 1935. He had refined and improved upon a procedure first performed in the early twentieth century by a German surgeon named Walter Kausch.

Dr L informed me that it involved the removal of my gall bladder, parts of my stomach and pancreas, and the duodenum, which is the beginning of the small intestines. Also to be removed would be a length of the small intestines and any affected lymph nodes. Thankfully, my liver was not affected. Once the resected tissues have been removed, the small intestines would be drawn up to be reconnected to the remaining organs.

The operation involved an open surgery with a cut across my abdomen. There would be several risks to bear in mind and these include excessive bleeding, leakages and other post operation complications. There would be considerable pain and I would be in intensive care for a couple of days. Recovery will take a few days and I should be able to be discharged a week or so after the procedure. His confidence for my recovery notwithstanding the complexity of the surgery gave me hope for a good outcome.

Dr D had also been around to explain other considerations related to the operation. In the event that when my abdomen was opened and it is found that cancer had spread elsewhere, the condition could be deemed inoperable. My wound would be closed up with no action taken. Under the circumstances, whatever tumours or cancer cells found would be left as they are and other treatment strategies would have to be instituted.

Dietary changes are important consequences of the Whipple procedure. As my digestive tract was affected, I would have to consume smaller meals but take them more frequently. The pancreas, which normally produces enzymes to help digestion may no longer do so and enzyme supplements would be required for every meal. The more severe concern is the pancreas' ability to produce insulin. Should this be affected there is an added risk of contracting diabetes. It was all beginning to sound quite ominous and challenging for a normal life ahead.

With the operation, there would be considerable stress. I would lose some weight and need to restore my strength as soon as possible. A high protein diet with supplements is a part of the daily fare. All these stipulations for food intake and nutrition are important to prepare for the next phase of my treatment. The body would take some five to six months to adjust to its new condition.

Upon my discharge, an oncologist would follow up with the treatment for cancer.

Settling In for the Operation

As the two weeks at home ensued, I tried to live as normally as I could under the circumstances. I drove to the nearby malls for our groceries and some meals. In many ways, these distractions helped to give me confidence that I would somehow be restored to a normal way of life.

Dr D made an appointment for me to be examined some ten days before the operation, on a Friday, 14th October. It was an assessment to ensure that I was physically fit to undergo the surgery as planned. My wife and son accompanied me for the examination and Dr D went over details of what was to come. He was very thorough and helpful answering any lingering questions we had.

I was pronounced both physically and medically fit for the surgery. I went home as mentally prepared as I could be for the operation to come. In the meantime we prayed and placed our trust in God.

I was readmitted on Sunday morning, 23 October, a day before the scheduled operation. As I settled into the ward, I was given instructions to prepare myself for the operation. It would be an early morning start. I was required to fast and clear all contents of my stomach later that evening. I was to have a good night's rest and be up early the next day. As I prepared myself for the next day's events, I continued to experience God's calm and peace.

It being a Sunday, visiting hours stretched the whole day from noon to just after eight in the evening. As expected, the ward was somewhat noisy with visitors. My wife went home to rest for the afternoon while my son came much later.

Shortly after three that afternoon, some of my fellow BSF leaders visited. I told them I was not anxious and trusted the Lord that all would be well. Matthew (a fellow BSF leader) then brought a wheelchair telling me that he was bringing me down for a walk and maybe coffee. As I arrived at the lobby, I came to realize that there were other fellow leaders assembling there. Led by our Teaching Leader (TL), the group had actually organized themselves to come pray with me and worship the Lord together. What a wonderful surprise.

As more leaders arrived, Matthew located a modest room interestingly marked "Quiet Room" at the back of the lobby. It was a room the hospital has very considerately allocated for visitors to spend quiet meditative moments on their own. The room was neutral in setting with a few colourful couches and simple chairs.

TL explained that we were gathered to worship the Lord and to pray for me. I had not been able to attend church for about a month and this was as close to a church service as I could get. I was moved by their show of love and concern. We sang a few hymns and TL shared from the Word of God. I could not remember the passage he read but whatever it was it edified me and we prayed. My choice for a closing hymn was *It is well with my soul,* which I felt expressed well my being at peace in the Lord.

We all sang the hymns, feeling the presence of the Spirit of God there that afternoon. It was an hour that overwhelmed me with the love and fellowship of this special group of brothers.

All of them came up to assure me that they would be praying for me through the day of the operation and through my recovery process. I am so thankful that I am part of a fellowship of men who love the Lord.

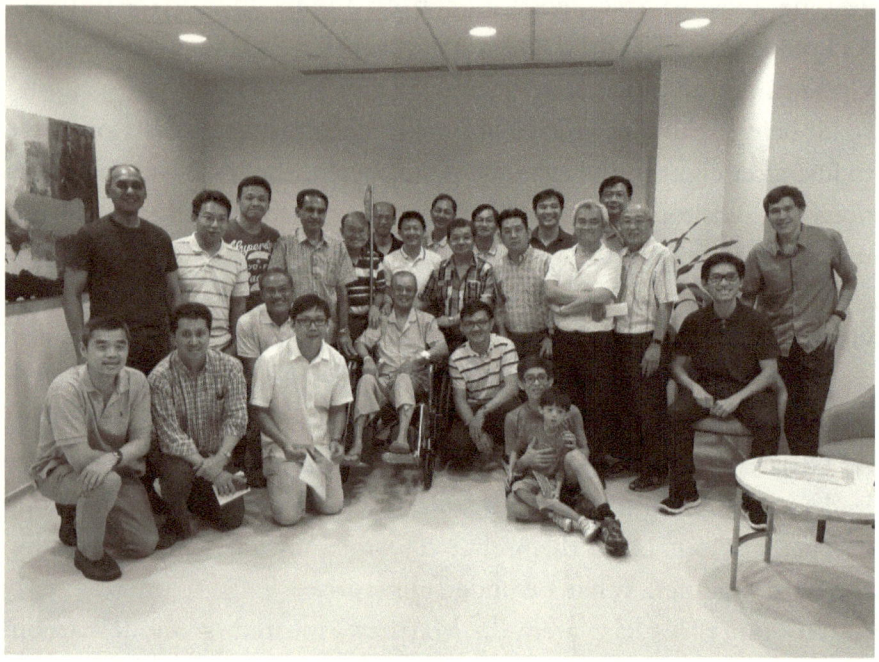

Pic 1: BSF Brothers at Prayer and Worship Service at NTFGH on 23 October 2016

As Matthew wheeled me back up to the ward, I watched some of them departing, and was glad that they could be with me in prayer and worship. BSF took on a whole new meaning for the term "Fellowship." We are indeed a family under God.

When my wife returned to learn of the service that was conducted specially for me, she too was overwhelmed and as visiting hours came to a close, we prayed for the operation the following day. None of us were anxious as we felt the Lord's presence. The lights were dimmed and I remembered drifting off to sleep.

Shortly before I slept, a nurse asked if I had medication from my family physician with me. They needed to record them prior to my operation. I called my wife and arranged for her to bring them early in the morning before my operation began.

I woke up early, perhaps just before six. I sat up briefly before going for a quick shower and donning a fresh set of clothes. It was around six-thirty when a porter appeared ready to wheel me to the theatre. I suddenly realized that my wife was making her way to the hospital and we would miss each other. In any case, my medication that was at home no longer mattered. I quickly borrowed a phone to call her. She was at the bus stop with her bus

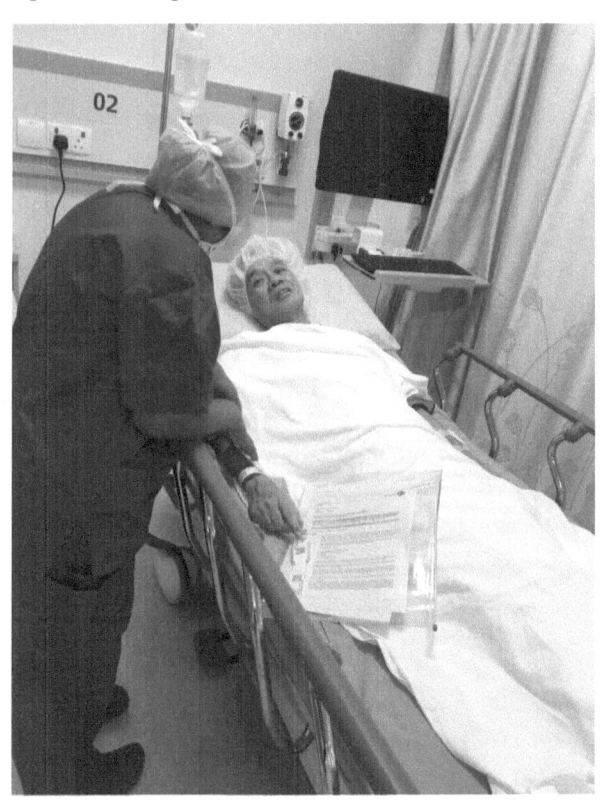

Pic 2: Being prepared for the operation

just approaching. I told her about being brought down to the operating theatre and that she need not come to the hospital. I had reached her in the nick of time so she did not have to make the futile trip. We praised God for His perfect timing.

The porter was ready and we set off on our little trip to the operating theatre. It was not even seven a.m. by the clock on the wall. Dr D arrived shortly thereafter and asked how I was. I thought I gave him a confident smile and he responded with a thumb's up indicating that all would be well. He was going to be part of the team performing my operation.

Kenny (a fellow BSF leader) arrived just as I was about to be wheeled into the theatre. With limited time, we prayed. He then took a couple of pictures of me to share them with the other BSF leaders. My operation was about to begin.

It was cold in the operating theatre as the anesthesiologist came up to greet me. Shortly after our conversation began a breathing mask was placed over my face and in no time I lost all consciousness. I only awoke from that deep slumber and came around some twelve hours later when all was over.

I slowly opened my eyes and saw the clock in the operating theatre showing that it was almost seven in the evening. I had been in OT for

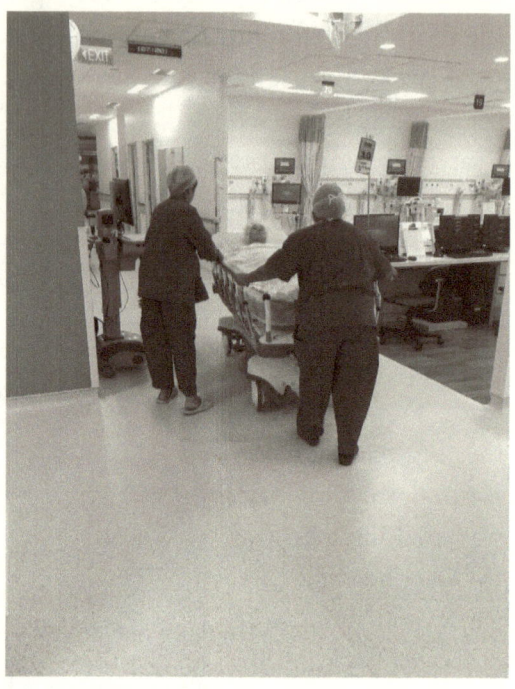

Pic 3: On the way to Operating Theatre No. 10

some twelve hours. The nurses were adjusting all the paraphernalia around me before moving me to the ICU.

Seeing that I was semi-conscious, they told me that the operation was over and that it was successful. I dozed off back into sleep.

At the ICU I was carefully transferred to a bed and connected up to another bank of equipment. It took an hour or so before all was done. A nurse told me that they had informed my wife that the operation was a success. The Lord had seen me through a long and difficult day.

*****

God's Faithfulness

One of my favourite hymns is *Great is Thy Faithfulness* written by Thomas Chisholm in the early part of the twentieth century. It was inspired by the passage in the Book of Lamentations (3:22-23) *"Because of the Lord's great love we are not consumed, for his compassions never fail. They are new every morning; great is your faithfulness."*

Chisholm lived a life that was ordinary, much of which was spent in poor health. In spite of the challenges, he went on to write some 1,200 poems and hymns, the most famous of which was *Great Is Thy Faithfulness*. The hymn was his acknowledgement of the unfailing faithfulness of a covenant-keeping God who gave him many wonderful displays of His providing care.[3]

God's faithfulness emanates from His love and compassion. *"Know therefore that the LORD your God is God; he is the faithful God, keeping his covenant of love to a thousand generations of those who love him and keep his commands."* (Deuteronomy 7:9). His desire was to restore mankind to Him after the Fall (Genesis 3). God's plan was one of redemption expressed through a man named Abraham with whom He established an unconditional covenant to bless him and the nations to come (Genesis 12).

God's Promise to Abraham

Abraham and his wife Sarah were both advanced in years. God, in keeping His promise, allowed Sarah to give birth to a son, Isaac. From Isaac came Jacob, whose name God changed to Israel. From Jacob came twelve sons who formed the twelve tribes of Israel.

God chose the Israelites to be His people to whom He revealed Himself and unfolded His plans. *"The Lord did not set his affection on you and choose you because you were more numerous than other peoples, for you were the fewest of all peoples. But it was because the Lord loved you and kept the oath he swore to your ancestors"* (Deuteronomy 7:7-8).

As the Israelites settled in the Promised Land, they sinned against God through their disobedience and worship of other gods. *"God found fault with the people and said: 'The days are coming, declares the Lord, when I will make a new covenant with the people of Israel and with the people of Judah"* (Hebrews 8:8)

The Westminster Confession explains "Man, by his Fall, having made himself incapable of life by that covenant, the Lord was pleased to make a second, commonly called the covenant of grace: wherein he freely offered unto sinners life and salvation by Jesus Christ, requiring of them faith in him, that they may be saved, and promising to give unto all those that are ordained unto life, his Holy Spirit, to make them willing and able to believe."[4]

The Israelites were punished for their sins. They were defeated in wars, captured and exiled. God in His grace and mercy however did not allow them to be totally destroyed. He preserved a remnant in order that Israel survived. So, from Abraham through the nation of Israel and the lineage of King David came another man named Joseph who was betrothed to the Virgin Mary. Mary divinely conceived and gave birth to Jesus that first Christmas night in Bethlehem some two thousand years ago.

Jesus, Son of God

The prophet Isaiah had foretold Jesus' birth, *"Therefore the Lord himself will give you a sign: The virgin will conceive and give birth to a son, and will call him Immanuel."* (Isaiah 7:14). God was revealing Himself progressively to the Israelites and to the world. He came in human form as Jesus that the world through Him will be saved.

Through His teachings and His works, Jesus revealed Himself as the Son of God and all those who believe in Him are forgiven of their sins. When Jesus shared His last meal with His disciples, He told them *"This cup is the new covenant in my blood, which is poured out for you."* (Luke 22:20). Jesus gave the wine and the bread at the Last Supper to His disciples to illustrate to them the symbolism of His sacrificial death on the cross. Christians today celebrate this sacrament as the Holy Communion in remembrance of His death for our sins.

Like the animals sacrificed for the atonement of sin, Jesus became the ultimate sacrifice by dying on the cross. Herein lies the new covenant of grace. *"This is the covenant I will establish with the people of Israel after that time, declares the Lord. I will put my laws in their minds and write them on their hearts. I will be their God, and they will be my people. ... For I will forgive their wickedness and will remember their sins no more."* (Hebrews 8:10, 12).

God's faithfulness is demonstrated through Jesus who came to save the nations from sin, both Jews and Gentiles, those who are not of Jewish descent. Redemption requires a price to be paid. That price was the blood of Jesus on the cross. God's covenant with Abraham was fulfilled. Through him, the nations are blessed. Jesus died so that we may be reconciled back to God.

Following Jesus' ascension to heaven, God gave us the Holy Spirit to indwell believers so that His presence is always with us. Jesus assured His disciples *"If you love me, keep my commands. And I will ask the Father, and he will give you another advocate to help you and be with you forever."* (John 14:15-16). The Holy Spirit is God in the third person of the Trinity. He is our helper, counselor and the Spirit of Truth within us. We receive the Holy Spirit when we accept Jesus as Lord and Saviour.

In God's covenant with Moses, the Israelites approached God through a high priest in the temple. Under the new covenant Jesus is our High Priest. We now approach God directly and personally without the need of an intermediary. We pray in Jesus' name *"... because Jesus lives forever, he has a permanent priesthood. Therefore he is able to save completely those who come to God through him, because he always lives to intercede for them."* (Hebrews 7:24-25)

Responding to a Faithful God

Because we have a faithful, promise keeping God, we can trust Him for all our needs. Our response to God's faithfulness must be one of obedience through our belief and faith in Jesus Christ. Oswald Chambers acknowledged "Faith is the entire person in the right relationship with God through the power of the Spirit of Jesus Christ."[5]

Thomas Chisholm in *Great is thy Faithfulness* demonstrated his trust in the sovereign God for all his needs. Reflecting on his own personal experience, inspired by the Holy Spirit, Chisholm wrote this refrain:

"Great is Thy faithfulness!" "Great is Thy faithfulness!"
Morning by morning new mercies I see;
All I have needed Thy hand hath provided —
"Great is Thy faithfulness," Lord, unto me![6]

*****

REFERENCES

1. Hruban, R. H. (2014). World Cancer Report 2014 - Pancreatic Cancer. World Health Organisation. Lyon Cedex, France: International Agency for Research on Cancer.
2. Mayo Clinic. (2017). Pancreatic Cancer. Retrieved March 14, 2017 from Mayo Clinic: www.mayoclinic.org/diseases-conditions/pancreatic-cancer/home/ovc-20268502
3. Gaither, B. (2017). Great Is Thy Faithfulness - The Story Behind the Hymn. Retrieved August 17, 2017 from Gaither.com: http://gaither.com/news/ "great-thy-faithfulness"-story-behind-hymn
4. The Westminster Confession of Faith. Chapter VII, 3.
5. Chambers, O. (1992). *My Utmost for His Highest*. Oswald Chambers Publications Association, Ltd.
6. Great Is Thy Faithfulness. Words: Thomas O Chisholm, © 1923, Ren. 1951 Hope Publishing Company, Carol Stream, IL 60188. All rights reserved. Used by permission. Reprinted under license #78637

5
PRAYING IN RECOVERY

*Do not be anxious about anything, but in every situation, by
prayer and petition, with thanksgiving, present your requests to
God. And the peace of God, which transcends all understanding,
will guard your hearts and your minds in Christ Jesus.*
Philippians 4:6-7

I Have never had a major operation before. In fact this was my first
experience of being hospitalised. In relating my medical history to
the medical team I had prided myself on being in excellent health all
these sixty-nine years of my life. My only previous encounter with a
hospital was a short afternoon surgery to remove a small cyst at the
base of my neck more than twenty years ago. It was benign and had no
consequential impact on my health.

Prayer Warriors At Work

While I was in the operating theatre undergoing the complex and
risky procedure, there was an army of prayer warriors praying for a
successful outcome. My family, my sisters, fellow BSF leaders, members
of our various churches and all our friends were praying ceaselessly.

They prayed for wisdom and guidance for the medical team, for
safety throughout the process and the recovery to follow. They prayed

for healing and a successful outcome. They prayed above all for peace and assurance of the Lord's presence for me and my family.

They prayed before the operation and throughout the day of the operation and the days following. This army of prayer warriors was with me throughout my journey.

At the ICU

I fell asleep quite easily once all the medical paraphernalia had been hooked up onto me at the ICU. I woke up only the next morning aware that my operation was all over.

The doctors and nurses examined me regarding my pain, my ability to feel, and my level of alertness and consciousness. Several times throughout the day I was tested to see if I could feel the sensations of touch and cold.

Pain management was an important part of the monitoring process and I was given some heavy doses of painkillers. One set of these painkillers was attached to bottles hanging by the sides of my body. The only pain I experienced however was when I asked to be turned onto my side. I could not move on my own and required the assistance of a nurse to do so.

I had nothing by mouth and all my nourishment was through intravenous feeds. As the hours went by, my lips were dry and began to hurt. To ease the discomfort ice cubes were rolled over my lips and momentarily placed in my mouth. It was a short but helpful relief.

My wife came by to visit that first morning, staying a while looking over me. I gave her a brief description of my condition regarding the level of pain and discomfort. She gave me her supportive looks and prayed silently.

My son and daughter-in-law, and my sisters came to visit sometime later. They were all glad and comforted to find me conscious and alert. God has seen me through the most difficult phase of the treatment process.

Every now and then the nurses would check on me and take note of my vital signs. With each change of nursing shift, they would surround my bed and briefed one another on my condition and the things to be mindful of. I lay motionless in bed listening to all that was needed to be done for me.

The nurses provided an extra pillow to help cushion the pain around my abdomen. One resourceful nurse constructed one out of two large towels folded into squares and encased them in a pillowcase. This helped a lot, as it was so much lighter and easier to handle.

Several times a day I would be asked to gauge the pain on a scale with ten being unbearable excruciating pain. Most times my record of pain would hover somewhere in the range of a five or a six. This allowed the medical team to regulate the amount of painkillers I needed.

Time to Exercise

Around the mid afternoon two visitors in white coats came to see me. They introduced themselves as the ICU's physiotherapists and they were there to make sure that I was able to exercise and move about. I was totally taken by surprise and protested that I was in no condition to do so.

The lead physiotherapist smiled and explained the importance of starting physiotherapy even in ICU. All they needed for me that first afternoon was to have me sit on a chair for an hour. I remarked that under the circumstances, it seemed too long for me to be up. They smiled reassuringly and said that if I was unable to fulfil the full hour they would gladly help me back to bed.

And so, with all my connections hooked onto movable poles, I sat up on a chair. It took a while to get everything in place and I was given every assurance that they would check in on me.

It was tiring and I tried to doze off as much as possible. Each time I opened my eyes to gaze at the wall clock it seemed to move ever so slightly. Finally, around the forty-five minute mark both agreed that I have done well for the day. They returned all my connections to their original positions and placed me back on the bed, promising to visit me again the next day.

God's Assurance of Care

Towards the late afternoon and early evening, another visitor surprised me. She introduced herself as one of the senior nursing staff and said that her father had asked her to visit me. Her father attends BSF and was one of those praying for me. Ms C explained that she works in ICU and was involved in the care plan for its patients. She reassured me that I was in a good condition and would look in on me from time to time. I thank God again that indeed, He sent fellow believers and angels to watch over me.

When my wife returned later that evening, I told her about the physiotherapists and Ms C. We chatted briefly about the experience that first day in ICU. We prayed and thanked the Lord for the care I received.

Sometime later, the doctor in charge of ICU came by. He was a tall and cheerful character who looked at me briefly and proclaimed that I was well, conscious and alert and should therefore not be at the ICU. He suggested promptly that I should be transferred to the general ward. I protested that I was just brought in the night before. He smiled, and before leaving told me that he would speak to my doctors and arrange for my transfer as soon as possible. As the lights were dimmed it was time to sleep. I was worn out by the day's activities having had only short stretches of sleep.

Early in the morning a new team of nurses took over and a new round of checks and examinations began. Two attendants greeted me and told me that they were there to clean me up and change my clothes. At the same time, the bed linen would be changed and all these would be done without my having to leave the bed. I was amazed how these were all done with great efficiency and care. I felt somewhat refreshed after a good wipe and noticed that my personal belongings that had been left in the ward had been brought to my bedside.

It was another day of "Nothing by Mouth" and there were ice cubes ready to soothe my dry lips and mouth. The nurses helped me turn onto my side every now and again to prevent me lying too long on my back. Pain was still manageable. My wife and son visited later that morning and I mentioned the possibility of my being transferred to the general ward. As usual we prayed together.

My two faithful physiotherapists returned about the same time as the day before. They were bright and cheerful and said that they would like me to exercise this time. All I had to do was take a walk from one side of my bed to the other side and back. It was to make sure that my legs could get the circulation they needed. After walking around the bed I would sit up again for another hour.

So once again we went about with all the instruments mounted on mobile stands. With each of them holding me on one side, I slowly walked from one side of my bed to the other and back. It was a short walk and I seemed steady enough under the circumstances. I sat down on the chair and was encouraged to try for an hour. As the hour approached, they congratulated me on my achievement and gently returned me to bed so I could rest again.

My wife returned early that evening and as we were chatting, Ms C came by to visit. I introduced my wife and we began a conversation about work at the ICU and onto the subject of church. As it turned out, Ms C attends the same church as we do. She is part of the music ministry and plays the piano for one of the services. God seems to be assuring us that we are in good familiar hands.

My final visitor is a doctor and one of the department heads. He was also attending BSF and was told that I was at the ICU. He knew my surgeons and was updated by them on my operation. We had a brief chat generally about my condition and how I was coping. I thanked him for his concerns and told him that I was very well looked after and truly appreciated the care and professionalism of the staff attending to me. To me he was another angel sent by God to bring assurance of His presence.

Transfer to the General Ward

It was close to eight o'clock when a nurse came into my room to inform me that I would be transferred to the general ward. I was surprised as there had been no indication of a transfer earlier in the day. I had now been in ICU for two days as initially planned.

An hour or so later, a bed was ready and the nurses started disconnecting the instruments monitoring me. I was slowly and carefully pushed out of the room, out of ICU, down the corridors and into a lift, to a ward on the twelfth floor. The bottles of painkillers were still hanging by my side and so were two bags that drained fluids from my abdomen.

The ward I was transferred to was similar to the one I was in for my previous admission for jaundice. This time my bed was the one facing the opposite direction but still beside the large window overlooking the shopping malls. It was refreshing to have a view of the world outside again.

As the nurses slide me onto my new bed, I quietly gave thanks to God for the quick improvement in my condition. I stayed briefly awake but soon dozed off.

The hospital informed my wife of my transfer and she in turn updated my BSF team and other friends of my situation the next morning.

I felt a great assurance of God's invisible hand working in my treatment and healing process. I had His peace and comfort during these difficult and painful days. Now that I was back in the general ward I would have the company of family and friends during visiting hours. They all came, happy to see that I was on the road to recovery, that the operation was a success and that God has been good. He answered our prayers.

*****

Praying for the Sick

Praying for the sick can be a challenge. Expectations are high and prayers for healing may not be answered the way we expect. Paul pleaded with the Lord, to no avail, to remove a thorn in his flesh. God's response was, *"My grace is sufficient for you, for my power is made perfect in weakness."* (2 Corinthians 12:9).

There can be joy for miracles and disappointments when healing does not come. Some may question the fervency of prayer, or the sufficiency of faith. Others question God. Few understand the sovereignty of God and His answer to prayers.

John Piper in his sermon *Christ and Cancer*[1] explains that God in His sovereignty allowed sickness and suffering to exist because of the "futility and corruption" of man's fallen world. Jesus has a ministry of forgiveness and healing though not everyone was healed. His was a "foretaste" of the final redemption to come. When Jesus returns, *"He will wipe every tear from their eyes. There will be no more death or mourning or crying or pain, for the old order of things has passed away."* (Revelation 21:4).

Piper believes that "We should pray for God's help both to heal and to strengthen faith while we are unhealed."[2]

Praying as a Body of Christ

In the Book of James, we are called to pray. *"Is anyone among you sick? Let them call the elders of the church to pray over them and anoint them with oil in the name of the Lord. And the prayer offered in faith will make the sick person well; the Lord will raise them up. If they have sinned, they will be forgiven. ... The prayer of a righteous person is powerful and effective."* (James 5:14-16). James called on the elders of the church to pray for the sick. The more we come together as a body of Christ, the greater is the unity of the body and the spirit.

Piper explains that the Apostle Paul also called upon others to pray for him when he was in trouble and in time of need. "If God is God, and it is his power that makes a difference in answering prayer, why does it matter how many people ask him? ... the more people there are praying for something, and thus depending on God for mercy and power, the more people will give him thanks and glorify him when the answer comes."[3]

James exhorts us to *"Therefore confess your sins to each other and pray for each other so that you may be healed."* (James 5:16). In confessing our sins we recognise our sinful ways and our need to change. This helps remove grudges or hurts that may have been the cause of our pains and aggravation of our sickness. Praying for each other therefore includes prayers of forgiveness and reconciliation.

God's Miracles

Yes, we should be praying for healing and even for miracles, those that may not have humanly logical explanations because *"with God all things are possible."* (Matthew 19:26).

C. S. Lewis noted, "A miracle is emphatically not an event without cause or without results. Its cause is the activity of God: its results follow according to Natural law. ... Nature is ready. Pregnancy follows, according to all the normal laws, and nine months later a child is born."[4]

In the light of C. S. Lewis' explanation, medical advances are God's miracles in our modern times. God's inspiration allows for the medical discoveries we have today. The dead may not have been raised in the spectacular fashion that Jesus did with Lazarus (John 11:38-44), but we are seeing the sick recover and life extended by the effects of modern medical science. These are God's miracles happening each and every day.

In the application of faith and prayer we should not ignore God's medical miracles. Martin De Haan recounts a sad story by Dr Paul Brand in the November 25, 1983 issue of *Christianity Today.* A 15-month old child died when his family depended solely on prayer presumably refusing medical treatment. The cause of death was meningitis, an ailment that could have been easily treated.[5] This was certainly not a case of the lack of faith or the fervency of prayer. This sad episode underscores the need to understand and appreciate that God brings together a number of resources to bring healing to us.

When God Calls Us Home

As mortals there will be a time when our lives come to a close. For Christians, it would be time to return home to the Lord.

In my elder sister's final days, we could only watch her manage pain under palliative care. It was a difficult time. Our prayer then was for the Lord to take her home. When she passed on, she was fully healed and restored by Jesus in heaven. Her pains and sufferings were over. We found comfort in Psalm 23. On her resting place is the verse *"Surely your goodness and love will follow me all the days of my life, and I will dwell in the house of the Lord forever."* (Psalm 23:6).

Paul tells us *"Do not be anxious about anything, but in every situation, by prayer and petition, with thanksgiving, present your requests to God."* (Philippians 4:6). As we pray, we surrender our anxieties and fears to the Lord. He is in control. Give thanks for the things that are around us, our family and friends. *"And the peace of God, which transcends all understanding, will guard your hearts and your minds in Christ Jesus."* (Philippians 4:7)

Personal Prayers

In Psalms 103 and 91, I found assurance in His promises and in His love. For peace and comfort I looked to Him in Psalm 23. He is my shepherd. I praise God for who He is and give thanks for each new day, and for the love and support I received.

I pray for wisdom and guidance for the medical team looking after me. I pray for healing, physical comfort and peace. I pray for forgiveness for things done that do not glorify Him. I pray for a closer walk with Him. I pray for my family and friends who are in turn praying for me.

I recently discovered *Mi Sheberakh* a Jewish Prayer for the sick.[6] It is normally prayed in the synagogue when the Torah is read. It is a prayer that is prayed over oneself or on behalf of another. It is good to pray for the sick. Take a look at it at: http://www.myjewishlearning.com/article/mi-sheberakh-may-the-one-who-blessed/.

*****

REFERENCES

1. Piper, J. (1980, August 17). *Christ and Cancer.* Retrieved September 9, 2017 from DesiringGod.org: http://www.desiringgod.org/ messages/christ-and-cancer

2. Ibid

3. Piper, J. (1996, January 7). *Prayer Changes People's Will.* Retrieved September 15, 2017 from Desiringgod.org: http://www.desiringgod. org/messages/prayer-changes-peoples-wills

4. Lewis, C. S. (2012). *Miracles* (C.S. Lewis Signature Classics Edition ed.). London, UK: HarperCollins. p 94-95

5. De Haan II, M. R. (1989). *Does God Want Me Well.* Grand Rapids, Michigan, USA: Radio Bible Class (Our Daily Bread).

6. Weintraub, S. Y. (2017). *Jewish Prayer for the Sick: Mi Sheberakh.* Retrieved September 16, 2017 from My Jewish Learning: http://www.myjewishlearning.com/article/ mi-sheberakh-may-the-one-who-blessed/

6
ROAD TO RECOVERY

Peace I leave with you; my peace I give you. I do not give to you as the world gives. Do not let your hearts be troubled and do not be afraid.
John 14:27

It was still dark outside. By the activities in the ward I guessed it was just after six in the morning. I was half awake and would intermittently fall back to sleep.

The nurses were already going about their chores. The breakfast trolley was coming round but I was still on "Nothing by Mouth." This was only the third day after my operation and I would need time for my digestive system to recover. I was very tired and unable to move much. Pain was manageable and that pillow over my abdomen appears to be effective as a simple pain absorber.

Dr D and Dr P came around to examine me that morning. They looked at the wound across my abdomen and observed that it was healing well. Dr L had decided on a single vertical cut from my navel to just below my chest instead of a long cut horizontally across the chest. That vertical cut was shorter and neater to facilitate healing. I was healing well and looked good from the effects of the operation. The doctors gave me words of encouragement before leaving to see their next patient.

Resting and Recovering

I thought that it would take a week or so for the wound to gain some basic healing. There were still risks involved and we needed to be cautious with all movements. That week after the operation was critical as any problems arising would usually have surfaced within those few days.

Much of my time that week would be spent just resting to let my body heal. I did not have the strength to do anything else. My extended quiet time with the Lord was very limited. I was in no position to read my Bible and managed a few short silent prayers.

My wife and I decided that I was not ready for visitors other than the immediate family. I was particularly delighted to see my grandson again when he came and greeted me. He was such a joy to have around and a boost to my spirits. We sent a few messages to my anxious friends updating them on my condition and advising against any visits in the coming days.

I was able to sleep through much of the day and awoke only when the doctors or nurses examined me, or when my family came to visit. By Friday evening my second full day in the general ward, I was feeling much better and sat up with the bed tilted at an angle. Much of the pain seemed to have subsided. I was still fed intravenously.

My doctors came round to visit and were pleased with my progress. There were no complications and they informed me that they had removed all the tumours and cancer cells visible during the operation. The Whipple procedure was completed as planned. It would take a while for my body to heal and I should be able to progress to some semisolid food within a couple of days. I thanked them for the good job they had done and appreciated their on-going care. Their report was encouraging and I gave thanks to the Lord for a successful operation.

It was now four days since my operation. I was beginning to feel a little more comfortable. We decided that my friends could visit from Sunday giving me an extra day to recover. Many were looking forward to seeing me again. It would have been almost a week since my operation.

Nursing Care

Deepavali, the Hindu Festival of Lights, arrived that Saturday. I greeted the Indian nurses attending to me. They appreciated the gesture and one or two said that they were from India and missed the celebrations at home. These are among the many nurses who are foreigners working at the hospital.

I have come across Malaysians, Filipinos, and Chinese from the PRC in the ward. They are easily identified by their accents and the way they speak. I was impressed by how friendly they are and believe their culture makes them so. Regardless of their nationality, they were dedicated and very professional in their duties. Thankfully, our Singaporean nurses and staff at the hospital are just as friendly, courteous and efficient.

I cannot help but appreciate how a culture of respect, friendliness and helpfulness will lift an organisation's level of efficiency and productivity. I graded NTFGH very highly for their standard of care and patient relationship. It works both ways. A smile, a compliment, a word of appreciation and a greeting to start the day all help make a demanding job more pleasant and satisfying.

Earlier in the day, my intravenous drips were taken off and I was placed on a soft diet. It was good to be able to eat again. I was feeling a little stronger and able to turn slowly on my side by myself. I was surprised and delighted by my ability to do so.

Glad to See You Again

That evening, I scanned my phone and saw the many messages of prayers and encouragement sent over the past week. I took some time to reply thanking everyone and updating them on my condition. Many were delighted to hear from me and responded immediately with thoughts of visiting in the coming days.

On Sunday, my old friends from school and my brothers from BSF were among my first visitors. We were glad to see each other and know that the Lord had answered our prayers.

Over the following days, other visitors included friends from church. One of them works at the hospital and visited several times. Her children even drew me a large get-well card that touched me immensely.

As the week passed, I showed signs of making good progress. The doctor in charge of pain management assessed that I no longer needed the painkillers. The two bottles attached to my abdomen were removed on Monday and I was left with only two other bags draining fluids from my internal organs.

My faithful physiotherapists had not forgotten me either. On my first day in the ward, they got me to walk from my bed to a corner on the opposite side. Progressively the distance increased and by the beginning of the following week I was walking out to the visitor lifts. It allowed them to gauge my gait and confidence moving around. I felt good and appreciated their efforts.

I was just so touched by all my many visitors and well wishers. Some came with gifts and flowers. It was a humbling experience. God opened my eyes to the love of both friends and family in a way I could never have imagined. More so, it was His love for me that affirms my faith in Him.

There was much prayer and there was much thanksgiving. We were all thankful for the progress I made and for the challenges overcome each day. I drew ever closer to God. Trusting Him became real.

Ready For Discharge

By early November, my condition improved significantly enough for the doctors to consider discharging me so that I could continue my recovery at home. My condition had stabilised.

There was general amazement at the speed of my recovery. When told of my pending discharge, some of my friends were surprised. The Whipple procedure was one known to take a much longer time to heal. That I could be discharged within such a short period after the operation points to miraculous healing.

Dr D was confident that I would recover well. On Tuesday, 1st November, he brought some interns to examine me. Together they removed half the staples holding my wound together. I was amazed that they did it quite painlessly. Next they removed the two bags that were draining fluids from my body.

By all measures, I have recovered well. I was strong enough to push myself up on the bed and to turn around onto my side. I could walk steadily and confidently. The only remaining concerns were my appetite and weight lost. These would require time to improve.

Dr D confirmed that I could be discharged within a day or two. It would be good for me to rest at home. I only needed to return the following week for a review and the removal of the remaining staples. There was not much else that I needed by way of treatment at the ward.

C, the dietician made an appointment to discuss my dietary requirements. He was a friendly young man armed with a stack of information on nutritional values and charts on different types of food. As I had lost a considerable amount of weight, the advice was for me to have a high protein diet supported by supplements.

C was particularly insistent that I must regain weight and body mass to be able to withstand the stress from the coming treatment for my cancer.

My eating habits had to change. I should have small meals, eating slowly and not rushing through the food. I was encouraged to eat and snack frequently. C remarked that I do not have too many dietary restrictions except to avoid deep fried and oily foods. My diet, he added, is a dream diet, something he was unable to recommend to other patients such as those with diabetes.

As my discharge became imminent, my wife packed some of my belongings for home that evening. I messaged my friends regarding my pending discharge in case they planned to visit.

On the morning of Thursday, 3rd November, Dr D came round for a final examination and review. He was pleased and informed me that I would be discharged that day. I had been in hospital for twelve days, and it was only ten days since the operation. It was indeed a miraculous rate of recovery and I can only ascribe it to God's invisible, sovereign hand. I looked forward to being home.

As the paperwork was being prepared, I was given some instructions on cleaning and dressing the wound and general care pointers for me at home. Shortly after lunch I was cleared to go. I changed into my street clothes and made a final check to make sure I had left nothing behind. It was time to thank the nurses and bid them and my fellow patients goodbye. We exchanged wishes for our speedy recoveries.

With a couple of small bags in hand, my wife, our son, and I made our way to the lifts. We went to the exit gates, scanned our passes and were out of the wards.

Arthur, my brother-in-Christ from BSF volunteered to drive me home. Waiting at the pharmacy, he glanced up and saw us approaching. He was amazed to see me walking steadily and confidently. It did not seem as though I had been through a major medical procedure. He half expected that I was coming down in a wheelchair, as most patients would require. I smiled and said that it was all about God, not me.

We collected our medication and headed towards the car park. Just as we approached the lifts, out came an elder from my son's church. He was with his wife about to visit me in the ward. They were very surprised and delighted to see me being discharged and on the way home. We spent a few moments in conversation at the lobby before proceeding towards Arthur's car. It was again God's perfect timing at work.

Looking back it would have been difficult for me to have the sense of confidence and peace I had, if not for the prayers and the knowledge of God's presence. He was there throughout for me.

*****

God's Peace

As I prayed for God's peace my thoughts wandered to the peace that I truly desired. The peace I imagined and sought would not be unlike the quiet and calmness described in Psalm 23: *"He makes me lie down in green pastures, he leads me beside quiet waters, he refreshes my soul."*

(Psalm 23:2-3). It is an idyllic peace that is from and rests on Jesus and is directed by Him.

Peace in the ordinary sense of the word suggests an absence of conflict. This is true for we should seek to have no conflict with anyone. Let the anger of the past be resolved just as Jesus taught us to pray *"And forgive us our debts, as we also have forgiven our debtors."* (Matthew 6:12).

Paul refers to God as *"The God of peace."* (Romans 15:33, Philippians 4:9, 1 Thessalonians 5:23), and says Jesus Himself is our peace (Ephesians 2:14). To the Philippians he wrote *"And the peace of God, which transcends all understanding, will guard your hearts and your minds in Christ Jesus."* (Philippians 4:7). God's peace is beyond our comprehension. At the centre of it all is Jesus Christ our Lord and Saviour.

Our Source of Peace

Jesus told His disciples *"Peace I leave* with *you; my peace I give you. I do not give to you* as the world gives. Do not let *your hearts be troubled and do not be afraid."* (John 14:27). Jesus' assurance of peace came in the midst of comforting His disciples as He was preparing to go to the cross. It was a difficult time with the disciples, confused and uncertain of what was to come.

There was a close and intimate relationship between Jesus and His disciples. Jesus had earlier washed His disciples' feet as a mark of their sanctification (John 13:4-10). He offered the bread and the wine taken in remembrance of Him as symbols of His body broken and His blood shed to take the penalty for their sins (Matthew 26:26-28). He promised them that He would return and to take them to where He would be going (John 14:3). He promised them the Holy Spirit (John 14:15-17). He promised them eternal life (John 14:19).

The peace of Jesus is one that comes out of an intimate relationship with Him. It is about being with Him and having the Holy Spirit indwell us, bringing us closer to God. James, tells us to *"Come near to God and he will come near to you"* (James 4:8).

Gary Burge explains in his commentary, "'Peace' refers to the Hebrew greeting *shalom* and for Jesus, refers to the aim of His work on earth: to restore the equilibrium and richness of humanity's relationship with God (Romans 5:1). Nothing in the world can offer such a gift. Jesus' *shalom* not only brings an end to the brokenness caused by sin, but it will be the fruit of the Spirit given when He departs."[1]

"But the fruit of the Spirit is love, joy, peace, forbearance, kindness, goodness, faithfulness, gentleness and self-control. Against such things there is no law."(Galatians 5:22-23). These gifts are priceless for in them we find the basis for our conduct, our relationships and peace. Anything contrary to these is to have our temperaments changed, relationships questioned, and to invite strife into our lives. Jesus' peace deals with our character and very relationship with God.

J. Keathley drew attention to Paul's letters that began with the greetings "grace to you and peace." Keathley explains that by doing so, Paul brought attention to the "unmerited blessings" and "saving relationship with a holy God" through Jesus Christ. "Grace always brings benefits and one of these benefits is reflected in the word 'peace' … Until we know and appropriate grace, we can't experience peace."[2]

Our Desire For Peace

It is difficult to deny that each of us has a desire for peace. Parents with young children may seek the peace and quiet of a home without boisterous kids. Those at work may long for peace from office politics and the stress of career demands. Those who are unwell would seek peace and comfort from anxiety and pain. Whatever our desires and demands, peace can appear elusive, fleeting and at times difficult if not impossible.

Peace in the context of our daily lives will require us to pause, to turn our minds away from the noise and the hustle and bustle of daily work, to set aside our anger, stress, fears and anxieties. We need solace and quiet, to calm ourselves and be alone. These are the moments to turn to our source of peace, Jesus Christ. These are the moments we seek Him in prayer and to hear His voice. The Psalmist says *"God is our refuge and strength, an ever-present help in trouble. … 'Be still, and know that I am God'"* (Psalm 46:1, 10). Jesus hears our prayers and intercedes for us. He is omniscient, fully aware of our needs.

Joy and Peace

It is interesting that love, joy and peace are gifts appearing in that order (Galatians 5:22). Does this suggest that one is the result of the other – that love leads to joy resulting in peace?

Jesus commands us to *"Love one another. As I have loved you"* (John 13:34). This is not an option. Love is both an act as well as an emotion. Joy would certainly be a result of one's act of love. Having joy reflects a state of peace in one's heart and in relationships with others. Having peace naturally brings joy to each of us.

Pastor John Piper explains, "peace happens when anxieties are removed. Peace is the condition of the heart when anxiety and fear and conflict are not troubling the heart. And, of course, this feeling is a good one. One could say a joyful one. ... Joy, however, is a much larger word, because the good feeling of joy that comes into the heart doesn't just come from the absence of worry or conflict. It comes from other things too, like 3 John 4 says: 'I have no greater joy than to hear that my children are walking in the truth.' Or James 1:2, 'Count it all joy when you meet various trials.' Or Romans 5:2, 'We rejoice in the hope of the glory of God.' ... So joy is a good feeling in the heart that is based on a much wider range of good things than peace is. But they are so interwoven that there could be no true heart experience of Christian joy without the heart experience of Christian peace."[3]

It is therefore no coincidence that Paul, as a preface to his call to pray with thanksgiving, tells the Philippians to *"Rejoice in the Lord always. I will say it again: Rejoice! Let your gentleness be evident to all."* (Philippians 4:4). Pastor Christopher Seah reminds us that this is a "commandment to be happy in the Lord. ... It is to rejoice in what He has done for us. ... We must not doubt God wants us to draw happiness from Him."[4] And so, in these moments of rejoicing let your gentleness, another fruit of the Spirit, be displayed. From Nehemiah we learnt, *"for the joy of the Lord is your strength"* (Nehemiah 8:10)

God's peace thus comes with each of us being filled with the gifts of the Spirit. Its objective is to allow us to leave our worries and anxieties with Jesus and enjoy His presence, to place our trust in Him. By doing so we can rejoice and let His peace overflow in us. God wants us to secure our happiness from Him. His grace of forgiveness sets us free from guilt and hopelessness when sin entered our lives. All that stands between His peace and us is our calling out to Him. Jesus is the source of our peace. Shalom.

*****

REFERENCES

1. Burge, G. M. (2000). *John: The NIV Application Commentary.* Grand Rapids, Michigan, USA: Zondervan.
2. Keathley III, J. H. (2005, April 22). *Grace and Peace.* From Bible. org: https://bible.org/article/grace-and-peace
3. Piper, J. (2015, September 25). *What's the Difference Between Peace and Joy.* Retrieved September 21, 2017 from Desirunggod.org: http://www.desiringgod.org/interviews/ what-s-the-difference-between-peace-and-joy
4. Seah, C. (2016, January 17). *God the Lord Is My Strength - Rejoice in the Lord Aways.* From Providence Reformed Presbyterian Church: http://providencerpc.org/wp-content/uploads/20160117_notes.pdf

7

WISDOM AND GUIDANCE

Trust in the Lord with all your heart and lean
not on your own understanding;
in all your ways submit to him, and he will make your paths straight.
Proverbs 3:5-6

Opening the door into our apartment was such a joy to me. I was last home almost two weeks ago. I quietly appreciated being back after such a challenging time. I changed into my comfortable home clothes and went straight to bed. I would require some time for rest and recovery. I needed also to eat well to regain some lost kilograms.

The week at home was rather uneventful. I lay in bed most of the time getting up only for meals and other essentials. I did not seem to have sufficient strength for any extended activity. There was still discomfort around the abdomen although the pain had largely subsided. We decided that under the circumstances we should not have visitors until I grew stronger.

Meals at the hospital consisted largely of a choice between porridge or soft cereals with some equally soft vegetables or finely minced meat. For breakfast there was the choice of sandwiches. My meals at home were not very different. My appetite was not there and eating was slow and laborious. Much as I tried, my food intake was very limited. The week passed by rather quickly and I soon found myself back at the hospital.

Back to the Clinic

Dr P greeted me with a broad smile and said that I looked good. He examined me and told me I was healing well and there were no complications. He would arrange for a nurse to remove the remaining staples and I should be on the road to recovery.

The conversation then turned to my referral to an oncologist. An appointment was made for Tuesday, 22nd November, some two weeks away. He mentioned that there was high likelihood of my undergoing chemotherapy and with a reassuring smile added that I would benefit greatly from it. I thanked him for his advice and promptly moved into another room for my staples to be removed.

Alternative Treatments

My son and daughter-in-law resumed their research on cancer treatment and the options available. It was something they had commenced in earnest following my diagnosis. They studied the risks and side effects of each treatment protocol and the many independent reports available. Interestingly there is now a sizeable body of information and knowledge regarding natural and alternative treatments for cancer. Many involve herbs, fruits and vegetables to prevent or retard the growth of cancers.

A significant number of websites actively promote alternative approaches for the treatment of cancer. One of these was *Chris Beat Cancer*. This is by a young man who in 2003, at the age of twenty-six found himself diagnosed with Stage III colon cancer. He had his surgery but declined chemotherapy. Instead, he went onto a diet of juices, fruits and vegetables and overcame his cancer. [1]

My son bought me a book on cancer cure and prevention. *Anti Cancer – A new way of life* by Dr David Servan-Schreiber[2] was more than just an interesting read. The author is a professor of psychiatry who in the course of his research subjected himself to an MRI and accidentally discovered a tumour in his brain. He then went through a whole regimen of treatment that included surgery and chemotherapy. His treatment impacted him in many ways turning his attention to the clinical practice of medicine and active cancer research.

Dr Servan-Schreiber's views on treatment changed when he came across two different schools of medicine in Tibet while visiting Dharamsala in India. One was based on Western medicine and the other on traditional Tibetan medicine using plant remedies. He wrote of how our bodies' immune system can be strengthened to defend itself against cancers. "If certain foods in our diet can act as fertilizers for tumours, others on the contrary harbour precious anticancer molecules."[3] Dr Servan-Schreiber went on to describe various natural plant foods that contain good anticancer properties. As a psychiatrist he also noted that stress and other emotional factors are possible contributors to the growth of cancers.

Going Forward

Over the course of the week we discussed the various options for cancer treatment, one based on an anticancer diet and the other on established medical treatment like chemotherapy. There was a growing trend towards natural cures and away from treatments such as chemotherapy and its many side effects. A number of commentaries, from qualified medical practitioners and scientific researchers suggested that approval for natural cures have been blocked by powerful pharmaceutical interests because of threats to their revenues.

There is no doubt that our lifestyles, stress and other environmental factors are also major causes of cancer. What we consume as food is high on that list. My friends who enjoy their drinks will debate if alcohol is one of those to be added to the list.

In addition to all these, there were also recommendations to look into Traditional Chinese Medicine (TCM). TCM can be curative or a health enhancer bringing balance to the body's natural state. The latter like traditional chicken essences and herbal teas are to level out the "ying" and "yang" forces so as to maintain a healthy body.

Perhaps the most famous patient of pancreatic cancer was none other than Steve Jobs, the co-founder of Apple and inventor of the iPhone. Jobs was first diagnosed in October 2003 and pursued alternative treatments for some nine months before accepting his doctors' advice on surgery. One report suggested that the nine months cost him the opportunity of a curative treatment and prematurely ended his life.[4] Jobs passed away on 5th October 2011 at the age of fifty-six.

As we discussed the treatment options, we all agreed to wait for the visit with the oncologist and to listen to the recommendations to come. We prayed for wisdom and guidance for ourselves and for the doctors treating me.

Meeting My Oncologist

The appointment with the oncologist on 22 November was preceded by a full blood test before the consultation. We met Dr H the oncologist taking over my treatment. For the first time since my admission, I was formally told that I had pancreatic cancer. Her pronouncement gave finality to my diagnosis and left us all with no doubt of what I had and for treatment ahead.

My cancer was assessed as Stage IIB, which meant that it had not yet spread into major blood vessels. It had nonetheless spread to nearby lymph nodes.[5] Had my tumours not been discovered, it could have easily progressed to a Stage III or Stage IV within a matter of a few short months.

Dr H shared the importance of reinforcing the surgery with chemotherapy. This was to ensure that all the cancer cells in my body were destroyed. Other options such as radiation were ruled out as not being suitable.

Dr H proposed that I go for two concurrent courses of chemotherapy so as to ensure a better outcome. One course would be by injections to be administered weekly and the other an oral course that requires me to take some tablets daily. There would be a total of six cycles, each cycle lasting three weeks followed by a week's break. The whole course would stretch for a period of six months.

We enquired about the need for two courses and for them to be taken concurrently. She explained that although chemotherapy by injection was generally sufficient, research data shows that its effectiveness would be reinforced by the oral course. There would be side effects to be considered and the medical team would monitor my progress closely.

We were uncomfortable with the thought of having two chemotherapy drugs at the same time. Chemotherapy is highly toxic. It destroys both cancer cells and good cells along the way. I was unsure of the combined side effects. Dr H suggested that we talk it over as a family while she ordered a scan to ensure that the cancer had not spread to my bones.

Dietary Concerns

Our final stop that afternoon was with dietician C. He greeted us with a cheerful smile that helped changed the mood. C's office was adorned with plastic models of food similar to those displayed in a Japanese restaurant.

C's first remarks to me were filled with concern. I had lost more weight since my discharge. I told him of my lack of appetite and difficulty eating. C suggested ways to have small meals at more frequent intervals. He even suggested that I take a greater interest in food by learning how to cook my own meals. I looked at my wife and laughed saying something to the effect that the kitchen was her domain. C wished me well as we departed and made our way home.

I updated my prayer warriors on the consultations and reviews. They kept up praying with me. I thank God for each and every one of them.

Decision Time

As we talked over the proposed treatment plans, I was in favour of going ahead with chemotherapy but not with two doses running concurrently. I was troubled and shared my concerns with others in the family. Together we prayed for wisdom and guidance.

My son and daughter-in-law encouraged me to look into a diet based on a variety of anticancer foods. The overall condition of my digestive system weighed heavily on my mind. With my limited digestive capability my body may be unable to process the food that was supposed to nourish me. We agreed that a diet based approach should be complementary to conventional treatment.

My bone scan was done on the afternoon of 2nd December. We met with Dr H on the afternoon of 7th December. Thankfully the results of the scan were good and there was no sign of cancer spreading to my bones.

I told Dr H of my concerns with having the double dose of chemotherapy. She encouraged me to give it a try indicating that she would stop the oral dosage as soon as I was unable to cope. She then suggested that I start my chemotherapy immediately that afternoon. I was taken aback and protested that I was not mentally and physically prepared to commence right away. I was hoping to start after Christmas but she stressed the urgency for me to get going. We agreed that I could start the following week.

I went home feeling apprehensive. I have had a measure of the Lord's peace since I was first admitted and right through the operation. But now, there is doubt and discomfort. I felt unprepared. Over the next few days I slowly accepted the decision and resigned myself to proceed. We prayed.

We returned to the Cancer Centre the following week on Wednesday, 14th December to start my chemotherapy. I had my blood test and waited to see my oncologist. As we were called into the room Dr H was away and Dr A the visiting consultant, met me. He had seen my reports and knew my concerns. He examined me briefly and then to my surprise, told me that the oral dose of chemotherapy was being cancelled. I needed only to take the chemotherapy by injection starting that afternoon.

Hallelujah! Thanks be to God our prayers have been answered. God had worked quietly in the background without our knowledge. By my delaying the start of chemotherapy, I was spared going through oral chemotherapy. All our apprehensions were lifted and God demonstrated again that He was in control over timing and events.

Interestingly, my son's visa for the US was approved towards the end of November. It was conditional on his arrival in the States within a given deadline. We talked about his pending move and felt confident that all would be well. The Lord will see us through this season. We felt His peace.

As we waited outside the chemotherapy room, I had no idea what to expect. What lay ahead for me were six long months of chemotherapy. We have prayed again for His wisdom and guidance. There was evidence that He was in charge and I was in His good hands.

*****

God's Wisdom

The Bible tells us that God is our source of wisdom. Job explained, *"His wisdom is profound, his power is vast. Who has resisted him and come out unscathed?"* (Job 9:4).

The craftsmen building the Ark of the Covenant and the Tabernacle had *"the Spirit of God, with wisdom, with understanding, with knowledge and with all kinds of skills"* (Exodus 31:3). We are told *"God gave Solomon wisdom and very great insight, and a breadth of understanding as measureless as the sand on the seashore."* (1 King's 4:29).

Jesus *"was filled with wisdom, and the grace of God was on him"* (Luke 2:40). Paul *"wrote you with the wisdom that God gave him."* (2 Peter 3:15). God's wisdom is *"first of all pure; then peace-loving, considerate, submissive, full of mercy and good fruit, impartial and sincere."* (James 3:17). James encourages us that *"If any of you lacks wisdom, you should ask God, who gives generously to all without finding fault, and it will be given to you."* (James 1:5).

God's wisdom is more than just knowledge. It includes skills, insight, understanding and power. It reflects His love, compassion and mercy. It is applied fairly, impartially and sincerely in His common grace to all. Pastor Deffinbaugh writes, "The beauty of God's character is that each of His attributes compliments the other attributes."[6]

Finding God's Wisdom

"The fear of the Lord is the beginning of wisdom" (Proverbs 9:10). This *"fear"* is a Godly fear, a reverential fear, one which R.C. Sproul describes as being in awe, reverance and respect for a Holy God.[7]

While we find God's wisdom reflected in all the books of the Bible, there are in particular five books of the Old Testament that are classified as the Wisdom Books. These are the Book of Job, the Psalms, Proverbs, Ecclesiastes and Song of Songs.

Job, Proverbs and Ecclesiastes are often singled out as the three books focused on the theme of wisdom. And, in the New Testament, the Book of James is generally regarded also as a wisdom book.

The wisdom literature "is the conviction that God has spoken to reveal His character and will, and that such knowledge is the foundation for life to be lived as a creature made in His image in the world He has created."[8] Proverbs begins with an explanation of its purpose: *"for gaining wisdom and instruction; for understanding words of insight; for receiving instruction in prudent behaviour, doing what is right and just and fair; for giving prudence to those who are simple, knowledge and discretion to the young – let the wise listen and add to their learning, and let the discerning get guidance."* (Proverbs 1:2-5)

From Job, we get to understand the nature of suffering and the sovereignty of God. God allows for suffering to happen and it is in the nature of a faithful God to restore us to Him.

Ecclesiastes is admittedly not an easy book with its apparent contradictions and somewhat depressing thoughts. *"Meaningless! Meaningless!" says the Teacher. "Utterly meaningless! Everything is meaningless." What do people gain from all their labours at which they toil under the sun?* (Ecclesiastes 1:2-3). However, what is refreshing is that life is not lived apart from God. *"This only have I found: God created mankind upright, but they have gone in search of many schemes."* (Ecclesiastes 7:29).

Ecclesiastes concludes with a call to once again, return to God. *"Fear God and keep his commandments, for this is the duty of all mankind. For God will bring every deed into judgment, including every hidden thing, whether it is good or evil."* (Ecclesiastes 12:13-14).

Applying God's Wisdom

We seek God's wisdom through prayer and meditating on His Word. The Holy Spirit guides us as we search for answers to our questions and dilemmas. Time with God is therefore purposeful in that we will discover His will for us.

Decisions on treatment for cancers are such moments when sound advice is critical. As we seek the wisdom of God and search the Bible it is unlikely that words like chemotherapy or radiotherapy would be found. We are more likely to find words referring to the blind, the lame and to leprosy.

When reading the wisdom literature, Professor Longman of Westminster Theological Seminary cautions that they are not laws or promises but "general principles of godly living." He explains, "you can't achieve wisdom by learning a list of rules and regulations that work in each and every circumstance of life. The wisdom of the Bible presents *principles* (author's emphasis) of godly living and advocates a mindset from which we can apply them." We are to recognise "our circumstances from Christ's eternal perspective. We will then recognise that God is at work for our good in even the most tragic and difficult situations." [9]

In my condition, we prayed for wisdom. We sought the Lord to grant my medical team the wisdom to treat me. We looked for the provision of experienced and skilful surgeons for my surgery.

We prayed for guidance concerning chemotherapy. God knew our fears and anxieties. He allowed a delay in the start of my treatment. We simply sought a postponement and waited upon the Lord. *"Be still, and know that I am God."* (Psalm 46:10).

What we have applied is our understanding that God works through various individuals and directs events when we place our trust in Him. We received advice and counsel from medical professionals, encouragement from family and friends and above all, comfort from His Word.

From the Prophet Isaiah, I learn to *"Seek the Lord while he may be found; call on him while he is near."* (Isaiah 55:6). I am reassured as Isaiah declared *"but those who hope in the Lord will renew their strength. They will soar on wings like eagles; they will run and not grow weary, they will walk and not be faint."* (Isaiah 40:31).

Many a times I will not be able to understand or explain why events and circumstances are what they are. I believe that God is a wise God. *'For my thoughts are not your thoughts, neither are your ways my ways,' declares the Lord. 'As the heavens are higher than the earth, so are my ways higher than your ways and my thoughts than your thoughts.'"* (Isaiah 55:8).

*****

REFERENCES

1. Wark, C. (2017). *Chris Beats Cancer*. Retrieved June 17, 2017 from Chris Beat Cancer: chrisbeatcancer.com

2. Servan-Schreiber, D. (2011). *Anticancer - A New Way of Life*. London, England: Penguin Books Ltd.

3. Servan-Schreiber, D. (2011). *Anticancer - A New Way of Life*. London, England: Penguin Books Ltd. p 144

4. Wikipedia. (2017). *Steve Jobs*. Retrieved June 29, 2017 from Wikipedia - The Free Encyclopedia: https://en.wikipedia.org/wiki/Steve_Jobs#Health_Issues

5. American Cancer Society. (2017). *Pancreatic Cancer Stages*. Retrieved October 6, 2017 from American Cancer Society: https://www.cancer.org/cancer/pancreatic-cancer/detection-diagnosis-staging/staging.html

6. Deffinbaugh, R. L. (2004, May 18). *The Wisdom of God*. Retrieved October 3, 2017 from Bible.org: https://bible.org/seriespage/4-wisdom-god

7. Sproul, R. C. (2017). *Wisdom - Introduction to Wisdom*. Retrieved October 3, 2017 from Ligonier Ministries: http://www.ligonier.org/learn/series/wisdom/introduction-to-wisdom

8. Jackman, D. (2003). *Opening Up the Bible*. London, England: Hodder & Stoughton.

9. Longman III, T. (1997). *Reading the Bible With Heart and Mind*. Colorado Springs, Colorado, USA: Navpress Publishing Group.

8

FAITH, HOPE & ENDURANCE

We remember before our God and Father your work
produced by faith, your labour prompted by love, and
your endurance inspired by hope in our Lord Jesus Christ.
1 Thessalonians 1:3

As I turned to my collection of messages I realised that I had unwittingly created a journal for my whole treatment process. They provided details that I could share in a testimony. God by His grace and mercy allowed me now to testify to what had been a most difficult and challenging journey.

The Chemo Experience

Ahead of me are six cycles of chemotherapy. Each cycle consists of three sessions with a week's break. The whole course for me would stretch over six months.

My first chemotherapy ("chemo") session started with a briefing on precautionary measures required. This was mandatory as chemo is a toxic drug and its effects have serious implications on the quality of life.

As I laid back on the recliner, the intravenous drips were put in place and the medication started to flow. A saline drip would commence first followed by the chemo drug and then a solution to flush the line.

The last I suppose was to ensure that the chemo medication was fully introduced into my body.

Chemo turned out to be a tiring exercise. It was late afternoon when that first session ended. It had taken about two hours. I had seventeen more to go.

The experience of undergoing chemo is difficult to describe. Mental preparation is important so that chemo despite its negative reports can be accepted positively. The side effects of chemo are well known. It is a highly toxic drug that kills both cancer cells as well as good cells. It is not entirely a targeted treatment and some are more general than specific to the cancer it is designed to destroy. For all intents and purposes, for late stage cancer patients it is not curative but as my oncologist explains, it is meant to prolong life and provide a better quality to life. The latter is not always the case and the side effects degrade rather than provide that quality of life. When this occurs, it is better to enjoy life as it is for whatever duration there is left.

Chemo however has also proven effective in many cases. There are success stories and many cancer patients have overcome their trials and survived to see cancers destroyed or held at bay.

My chemo experience was not without its difficulties and side effects. The battle within me was being fought on several fronts. It was a battle of endurance and I needed all my strength not to be depressed or demoralised. It was a tiresome, painful, difficult and challenging process. My family and friends encouraged me to remain positive.

We had an additional weapon in the fight and that was to trust the Lord and place our hopes in Him. We prayed specifically for strength to endure the treatment process, for the Lord's presence to be with me. We prayed for wisdom and guidance for the medical team, and for His healing to be complete.

Keeping Up with God

Since the start of the New Year, I had decided to follow a programme on my online Bible to read the entire Bible in one year[1]. I took that as a personal commitment and discipline for my daily devotion. I started on New Year's Day and gladly maintained the schedule. I also followed a second online devotion with *Our Daily Bread*[2] to complement my Bible reading programme.

I was encouraged by the prayer support and inspirational messages received. Without the Word of God I could have lost hope and have no answers to the "what if" questions in my mind. I had Jesus' assurance: *"Do not let your hearts be troubled. You believe in God; believe also in me. … I am the way and the truth and the life."* (John 14:1,6). I felt Jesus' presence around me. I could trust Him. He is God, my Lord and Saviour.

Chemo's Progress and Side Effects

Side effects differ from patient to patient. My experience started with fatigue and lethargy. The fatigue crept up on me and stayed on for the few days after each session. Staying up and remaining alert was difficult. Eating became laborious. It would take me almost half an hour to finish a small bowl of oats.

The more difficult side effects came with my second cycle. In addition to the fatigue, the onset of aches and pains were just the start of the battle inside me. I felt pain starting in the shoulders and then spreading slowly to the elbows, arms, hands and parts of my legs. It made getting up, moving around and even having a meal a struggle. Lifting a toothbrush to brush my teeth was difficult. The pain affected my sleep and grew in intensity.

I called the Cancer Centre and sought advice from the doctors. Dr S examined me and tested me for several conditions but found nothing significant. The only possible explanation was the side effect from my chemotherapy. I was prescribed two sets of oral painkillers, one for a milder pain and the other to be taken when the pain got more aggravated.

Shortly after the start of the fourth session I developed a nauseous feeling. It welled up in me and I felt more uncomfortable as the minutes ticked by. The nurses kept a close eye on me. When I threw up, they rushed to help and the doctor on duty examined me.

Nausea became a constant reaction to my chemo in all the subsequent sessions. Back home, I felt better after a while, and did not vomit any more for the rest of the days ahead. The medication I took caused drowsiness and allowed me to sleep well through the night.

The second chemo session of the third cycle was probably the most difficult session I experienced to date. I felt the nausea from the start and all through the afternoon. I vomited twice at the end of the chemo and was probably dehydrated by then. I was administered an anti-nausea drug intravenously and prescribed a stronger anti-nausea medication to take ahead of the next chemo session.

My wife thought that I was intimidated by the thought of chemo. The fact that I vomited only at the chemotherapy centre and not at home suggested to her that my condition was more psychological than physical. I thought that it was more likely the smell I encountered. As I entered the chemotherapy centre that smell wafted into my nostrils and I had a distinct look of discomfort. A nurse agreed that there was a distinctive smell around the room which some other patients had also expressed their discomfort with. We prayed.

Completing my third chemo cycle was a significant milestone. This meant completing half of my chemo requirements and was an important psychological halfway point. As part of the midcourse review, I had a CT Scan and an electrocardiogram (ECG) to check my heart's performance. Thank God, there were no abnormalities. I prayed for strength to complete the whole course. I needed to endure and persevere with God's help.

The next chemo cycle would be done in the morning, at 9:00 am. I thought that would be good, as I needed only a light breakfast before chemo. I could eliminate lunch, hunger and delays as potential reasons for the onset of past episodes of nausea. The morning schedule for chemo would be a good test of my theories. The whole experience seemed better and I was home around noon. The day was done and I could rest. There was the feeling of nausea but no vomiting.

At the start of the fifth cycle I realised that there was a noticeable improvement to my appetite. I could now finish my meal within a reasonable time and with less effort. The recording of my weight at the centre registered a slight increase this week. It was good news.

Interestingly, even as I was slowly starting to eat better and beginning to enjoy food again I still needed to exercise caution not to over eat or eat too fast. With each meal I needed to take my enzyme pills to help digestion. Then there was also the occasional diarrhoea. I thought to myself, if it was not coming out from the top it was coming out from the bottom. I took my prescribed anti-diarrhoea tablets and prayed that the diarrhoea would cease.

On reflection I am grateful that I was spared other side effects like hair loss, mouth ulcers and skin rashes.

Christmas and Easter

Christmas and Easter came in the midst of my chemo sessions. Both gave me reason to strengthen my faith and trust in God's will and good purposes for me.

The joy of Christmas has always been about the celebration of the birth of Jesus Christ. God had come to earth in human form, born of the Virgin Mary, in a manger some two thousand years ago.

With Easter, I thought of Jesus dying on the cross as a sacrificial lamb to atone for our sins. It was by His death that my sins were forgiven and I am reconciled to God. What if there was no Jesus? What if there was no forgiveness of sin?

As I explored these all too familiar questions, I found no other source of assurance except to believe in Jesus. He is the Son of God sent to bring me salvation from my sinful ways and ultimate death. I could not think of another religion that spoke to me of a relationship with God as Father, and a relationship based on His love and compassion for mankind.

This Easter, I reminded myself again of the verse *"For God so loved the world that he gave his one and only Son, that whoever believes in him shall not perish but have eternal life."* (John 3:16)

Chemo Breaks

Chemo breaks were a great relief. The first break in early January was particularly significant as my son and family prepared to leave for the States. The day they left coincides with the last day of my chemo break. It was a nice coincidence and I felt strong enough to see them off with mixed feelings – sad that they were leaving as we would miss them. Glad though and thankful to God for the time they spent with us, time that allowed us to enjoy our grandson. We thank the Lord for His perfect timing allowing us to be together during my critical days in hospital. Now having seen me start on my chemo journey we have the confidence that all would be well.

Chemo breaks also allowed me time to try getting out of home for a change. We thought being out for a while might help. We would make our way to the neighbourhood mall for some groceries and a short walk. The excursions were not all that long, perhaps less than an hour but getting out refreshed me and I felt better.

The second cycle ended just two days before Chinese New Year. We were not ready for visitors and so had quiet time for ourselves. I did however miss the annual reunions but everyone understood my condition and wished me a speedy recovery in the midst of all the New Year greetings.

After my third chemo cycle, my friend Joe from primary school suggested visiting my old residence at Emerald Hill for old times' sake. We all practically grew up around that house and the neighbourhood. We decided to gather to celebrate my achievements with chemo thus far, and settled on the Friday evening of 3rd March.

It turned out to be a good reunion. There was close to a dozen friends waiting for me. They were all so glad to see me up and about. They told me I looked good and confident. It was, I said, all by the grace of God. It was a good evening out, lifting my spirits and giving me confidence that I need not be home bound by chemo and its side effects.

End of Chemo

May 2017 was significant as I marked my seventieth birthday. I thank God for the gift of life. My life is truly in God's hands and my hopes are anchored in Him.

Finally, the last chemo session arrived. I was back to having it done in the afternoon. As though it was a last opportunity for me to experience the effects of chemo, I had to feel nauseous again and for a grand finale, I vomited on the way out of the chemo centre. Thankfully, I had a plastic bag with me and did not mess up the floor. I felt better and we made our way to catch a taxi home. Oh what a relief! It is all over! My chemo, it is done!

We prayed and gave thanks to the Lord for seeing me through the entire chemo treatment. We thanked our friends and prayer warriors and hoped for healing to be complete in God's hands. I felt good and just wanted to rest and recover in the days and weeks ahead. It had been a long tiring and difficult journey.

*****

Christian Suffering, Faith and Hope

Cancer is such an overpowering disease that it strikes fear in those afflicted bringing the spectre of death, suffering and pain. The oft-asked question is why God allows diseases, tragedies and evil to exist. This is a difficult question and we may never truly know the answers on this side of heaven.

On Suffering

One of the best Biblical illustrations of suffering is to be found in a man named Job. The Book of Job describes him as one who *"was blameless and upright; he feared God and shunned evil."* (Job 1:1). Yet, God allowed Job's faith and obedience to be tested. Despite the tragic loss of his wealth and children, Job refused to curse God. Instead Job worshipped the Lord and said *"The Lord gave and the Lord has taken away; may the name of the Lord be praised."* (Job 1:21). Job in response to his wife's call to curse God and die asked, *"Shall we accept good from God, and not trouble?"* (Job 2:10).

Timothy Keller writes, "no matter what precautions we take, no matter how well we have put together a good life, no matter how hard we have worked to be healthy, wealthy, comfortable with friends and family, and successful with our career – something will inevitably ruin it."[3]

At a more personal level, one of the more difficult issues concerns the sovereignty of God. Pastor Derek Thomas posed the question, "Is God sovereign and in control but unwilling, or is He sovereign but not in control?"[4] God being sovereign obviously is in control and nothing happens outside His knowledge.

In truth, it is often difficult to make sense of our circumstances in the midst of suffering. We need to seek our comfort and peace in Jesus Christ. The Psalmist asks, *"I lift up my eyes to the mountains — where does my help come from? My help comes from the Lord, the Maker of heaven and earth."* (Psalm 121:1-2).

Billy Graham offers three attitudes to be adopted in the face of suffering. First is an attitude of worship and to place our trust in God. Second is an attitude for learning about God, others and ourselves so that we can minister under the circumstances. Finally, is an attitude to glorify God for Jesus is in control.[5]

God knows our our pains and sufferings. Keller states, "Only Christianity, of all the world's major religions, teaches that God came to earth in Jesus Christ and became subject to suffering and death himself."[6]

Faith and Hope In Jesus Christ

That we should place our faith in Jesus Christ, is to trust that He has our best interests at heart. We look to Jesus in the hope of a better day and a better outcome for our trials, challenges, pain and suffering.

Paul declared, *"we have been justified through faith, we have peace with God through our Lord Jesus Christ, through whom we have gained access by faith into this grace in which we now stand. And we boast in the hope of the glory of God. Not only so, but we also glory in our sufferings, because we know that suffering produces perseverance; perseverance, character; and character, hope. ... And we know that in all things God works for the good of those who love him, who have been called according to his purpose."* (Romans 5:1-4, 8:28).

R. C. Sproul explains, "Paul does not say here that all things that happen to us are good things. ... all these things that happen to us are working together for our good. ... these things are part of the Refiner's fire, the crucible of the kingdom of God."[7] We need to see God in all His sovereignty bring goodness in the face of our difficulties. These could well be testing times and training times to enable us to see and experience God's love and grace first hand.

Jesus' time here on earth was to minister and reveal God to us. The Book of Hebrews reminds us that *"we have a great high priest who has ascended into heaven, Jesus the Son of God, let us hold firmly to the faith we profess. For we do not have a high priest who is unable to empathize with our weaknesses, but we have one who has been tempted in every way, just as we are—yet he did not sin. Let us then approach God's throne of grace with confidence, so that we may receive mercy and find grace to help us in our time of need."* (Hebrews 4:14-16).

Hebrews Chapter 11 has a wonderful description of the Biblical men of faith. They trusted God, responded to His call yet many did not live to realise the objective of their calling. *"Now faith is confidence in what we hope for and assurance about what we do not see."* (Hebrews 11:1).

Our faith rests in the hope of a better future, one which is without the pain and suffering that we now experience. The Apostle John wrote of this hope and new life. *"'Look! God's dwelling place is now among the people, and he will dwell with them. They will be his people, and God himself will be with them and be their God. He will wipe every tear from their eyes. There will be no more death or mourning or crying or pain, for the old order of things has passed away.'"* (Revelation 21:1, 3-4).

Jesus' promise is that He will return to bring us there. *"My Father's house has many rooms; if that were not so, would I have told you that I am going there to prepare a place for you? And if I go and prepare a place for you, I will come back and take you to be with me that you also may be where I am."* (John 14:2-3).

Our faith and hope in Jesus Christ is therefore to be united in glory with God our Heavenly Father. This is the hope of restoration and reconciliation to our Father in heaven, with our bodies renewed.

*****

REFERENCES

1. Olive Tree Bible Software. (2017). *Bible By Olive Tree.* Retrieved October 10, 2017 from Olive Tree Bible Software: https://www.olivetree.com

2. Our Daily Bread. (2017). *Our Daily Bread.* Retrieved October 10, 2017 from Our Daily Bread: https://odb.org

3. Keller, T. (2013). *Walking with God through Pain and Suffering.* Petaling Jaya, Selangor, Malaysia: PVM Harvest Resources. p 3-5

4. Thomas, D. (2017). *The Book of Job.* Retrieved October 10, 2017 from Ligonier Ministries: http://www.ligonier.org/learn/series/the-book-of-job/

5. Graham, B. (2007, November 30). *Suffering: Why Does God Allow It?* Retrieved October 18, 2017 from Billy Graham Evangelistic Association: https://billygraham.org/story/suffering-why-does-god-allow-it/

6. Keller, T. (2013). *Walking with God through Pain and Suffering* (PVM Harvest Resources, Petaling Jaya, Selangor, Malaysia ed.). London, UK: Hodder & Stoughton. p 120-121

7. Sproul, R. C. (2003). *The Invisible Hand - Do all things really work for good?* Phillipsburg, New Jersey: P&R Publishing Company. p 171, 175

9
HEALED THROUGH FAITH

Lord my God, I called to you for help, and you healed me.
You, Lord, brought me up from the realm of the dead;
you spared me from going down to the pit.
Psalm 30:2-3

With the completion of my chemotherapy I had two weeks' break without any instructions on treatment or medication except those that prevent nausea, diarrhoea and pain.

I had no clue as to what to expect or what might be prescribed. I like to believe that God has healed me through faith. Going through chemo was probably one of the most difficult times in my life. Each time I sat on that recliner in the chemotherapy room and had the drips hooked up to me, there was a flood of mixed emotions. For the next two hours or so, I would be in a helpless state, at the mercy of the drugs slowly dripping into my body accompanied by some occasional pain. I have not actually heard of someone being "cured" of cancer but I have heard of remissions and take it to mean that the cancer remains but is no longer growing. Whatever those thoughts were, I would pray and leave it to God and His sovereignty.

The effects of chemo were uncomfortable to say the least. The fatigue and the lack of energy and strength left me lethargic and occasionally a little depressed. As for the pain, the nausea and the diarrhoea these were all managed through medication and they generally did their job.

Reliance on God

I am glad that in all those moments of doubt, helplessness and occasional depression, I had God to look to. I would say a short prayer and recall verses from the Word of God. My morning reading of the Bible was most helpful. Many a time, the passages I read spoke to me. Some lingered longer than others but that routine became an anchoring point each day. Then there were the prayers I said quietly prior to and often during each chemo session, they allowed me to place my hopes on Jesus.

Cancer is a long-term ailment that requires lifelong management and care. Thank God the rates and probabilities for survival are much better today than those in the past.

My family and friends were also delighted that my chemo was finally over. We continued to pray for good results, trusting that the Lord will heal me completely. I had the peace of the Lord and any initial fears and anxieties were no longer there as the days progressed.

Chemo's Toll

Chemo had taken a toll on me physically and psychologically. I thank God that the latter was not too difficult to overcome as I found assurance in the Word, and through the prayers and encouragement from friends and family. Physically I would need to improve on my appetite and try to restore my body and regain some weight lost.

Each day had become a standard routine of eating, sleeping with some reading or television. I am not a fan of TV and only watched the news channels and an occasional documentary. More often than not I would doze off in front of the TV only to be chased off to bed by my wife. Exercise was limited to walking around the apartment and occasionally around the void deck down on the ground floor. I now use a walking stick to allow me something to hold onto in moments of unsteadiness or tiredness. I had fallen twice in the weeks before when we returned home either from hospital or from an outing to the nearby malls. Falls can have severe consequences and are to be avoided at all cost.

End of Chemo Review

The end of May approached and on the morning of the 29th we made our way back to the Cancer Centre. I had several vials of blood extracted for tests before making my way to another CT scan. The following day would be the big one when we meet the oncologist for the results. Interestingly, I felt the peace of the Lord and gave no further thought as to the outcome of the morning's tests and scans.

The appointment with the oncologist on 30th May was at 11:30 am, late in the morning. I was now a familiar face and was directed to wait to see the oncologist. My wife was with me to hear the results. We had no expectations and prayed for the results to be favourable. I strode slowly into the clinic with my walking stick in hand. A young unfamiliar face greeted us, smiling broadly. He introduced himself as Dr S and seated us down.

The first words from Dr S were "I have good news for you." It was a declaration I had been hoping for but was not quite expecting. I think my wife and I were momentarily speechless and certainly overcome with both surprise and joy.

Dr S took us through the tests results. My CT scan was clear and excellent but my blood tests were the best results possible. One by one, he rattled them off – my cancer markers are at 10, meaning that there are no more cancer cells in my body. I am cleared of cancer!

I was more than speechless. I was more like, stunned! That was the best declaration I could have hoped for. It had not crossed my mind before that I could be totally rid of cancer. God, you are such a wonderful, majestic healer. There must have been tears welling up in my eyes. I think we did say aloud, "Hallelujah! Thank you, Lord!" not as an expression of relief but an expression of gratitude and joy. Dr S must have paused to allow that momentary burst of joy to settle in our hearts and minds before proceeding with the rest of his remarks.

Dr S then further explained the wonderful improvements I had made. He recalled that at the peak, my cancer markers exceeded 1000 and now having come down to 10, it was a remarkable change. At 10, I am in a normal state. He mentioned that only some ten per cent or less of cancer patients with my condition achieved such results. I knew it was God's miraculous healing work.

As my euphoria calmed down, Dr S then cautioned that pancreatic cancer is known to be aggressive and may recur. I should therefore continue take the necessary precautions and monitor my condition regularly. I would be required to return every three months for a full blood test, and a CT scan every six months. He advised that other than that, I was to go enjoy myself and make the best of the time I have. The first question on my mind was whether I was fit to travel. "Certainly, please do so," he smilingly replied and added that we should do so as soon as we can. He asked if we had any thoughts on where we wanted to go, and we answered, "to the States to visit our grandson." He laughed and gave us his full permission to go ahead.

All other indicators from the tests were well within the normal range. My kidney functions, my thyroid, my cholesterol and sugar levels were all good. My blood pressure was normal and there was no sign of diabetes. My pancreas' ability to produce insulin had not been affected. My liver was also functioning well. Dr S was certainly as happy as we were. His broad smile and tone affirmed our relief and gave us every confidence for life to return to normal.

We thanked Dr S for sharing the results and advice with us and for the medical team that took such good care of me. To the nurses, we wanted to thank them and express our appreciation for their dedication and excellent care. As we take our leave from the Cancer Centre we were overwhelmed by what we had just heard. I could not be more excited to get home and share the good news with all our family and friends, especially all my prayer warriors who had been so faithfully praying for me. God has answered our prayers and all glory be unto to Him. Amen.

We prayed and gave thanks to God for His healing powers. All the events that went by these past eight months could not have come to such a wonderful conclusion if not for Him. Jesus was there with all of us when we prayed and called for help.

My prayer warriors had prayed faithfully in the belief that God answers prayers. I thank God for each and everyone who stood with me through this tumultuous period. I could not wait to send a message to all to share the good news. My message was short and simple. It informed everyone that I was cleared of cancer with my cancer marker falling to just 10 from over 1000. All my blood test results were normal and I had no signs of diabetes. I thanked God and each and everyone for keeping me in prayer and proclaimed God to be my healer.

Almost immediately after I sent the message, my phone buzzed with pings as messages from my chat groups came flooding in. It went on almost continuously for a good fifteen minutes or so and continued on throughout the day. Without exception, all expressed their joy and congratulated me on overcoming one of life's greatest challenges. For the next few hours we just kept thanking God for this wonderful miracle.

I spent the rest of the day just resting in the peace of the Lord. I think we sang softly a few hymns of praise and just soaked in God's goodness and love. I do not think I had a day such as this for a very long time. I thank the Lord for His gift of new life.

Sharing My Testimony

I conceived the idea of writing a book regarding this episode in my life sometime at the end of March or early April. I was then still going through my chemo. I shared the idea with my family and they encouraged me to do so.

As it was, I did not yet know the final result of my treatment but I felt that whatever the outcome, I had already enjoyed the grace of God. Jesus was undeniably there for me over the preceding months through my treatment. For whatever the final outcome, I wanted to glorify Him with my story. It would be an act of appreciation for all my friends and family members who stood with me. Moreover, I would be able to record my thanks and appreciation to the medical team and staff of NTFGH.

Towards the end of May when chemo was all done, I again gave serious thoughts to this book. The news of being cancer free increased my motivation and gave me greater impetus to completing it. Now I have an additional objective for this book and that is to encourage those going through cancer to place their hopes in our Lord Jesus Christ. I have been healed by God through faith and prayer. It would be great if my story allows others in similar situations to have a relationship with Jesus and to anchor their hopes in Him. Sole Deo Gloria.

*****

Soli Deo Gloria – To God Alone Be the Glory

Five hundred years ago on 31ˢᵗ October 1517, Martin Luther an unknown monk nailed his Ninety-five Theses on the door of his church in Wittenberg, Germany, questioning the prevailing practices of the Roman Catholic Church. This sparked the Protestant movement that became known as the Reformation. The "Five Solas" in Latin girded the Reformed church that emerged from the Reformation and became the focus of their theological message.

Scripture alone *(Sola Scriptura)* underscores the authority of scripture in the teachings of the church. Justification, the declaration that sinners are righteous before God, is because of Christ alone *(Solus Christus)*, by grace alone *(Sola Gratia)* through faith alone *(Sola Fide)*.

The late James Montgomery Boice, senior minister of Tenth Presbyterian Church in Philadelphia wrote "… each of the other solas leads to the last and final sola, which is 'to God alone be the glory.' That's also the final point of Romans 11:36, which concludes with the words: 'to Him be the glory forever! Amen.' When we ask why that should be, the first part of the verse is the answer. It is because all things really are 'from Him and through Him and to Him.'".[1]

Expressed in the five solas, the Reformation brought back the centrality of God's glory in *Soli Deo Gloria*.

What is God's glory?

Moses asked the Lord to show him His glory. *"And the Lord said, 'I will cause all my goodness to pass in front of you, and I will proclaim my name, the Lord, in your presence. … But, he said, 'you cannot see my face, for no one may see me and live.'"* (Exodus 33:18-20).

When Jesus was born in the manger in Bethlehem, Luke tells us *"Suddenly a great company of the heavenly host appeared with the angel, praising God and saying, 'Glory to God in the highest heaven, and on earth peace to those on whom his favour rests.'"* (Luke 2:13-14)

God's glory appears from all His goodness, His holiness and His name. The prophet Isaiah proclaimed *"Holy, holy, holy is the Lord Almighty; the whole earth is full of his glory."* (Isaiah 6:3). It is on account of His holiness that Moses or any of us is not allowed to see God's face.

We see God's glory in His name *"Ascribe to the Lord the glory due his name; worship the Lord in the splendor of his holiness."* (Psalm 29:2). *"Lord, our Lord, how majestic is your name in all the earth! You have set your glory in the heavens."* (Psalm 8:1).

When God called Moses at the Burning Bush He said, *"I am who I am. … This is my name forever, the name you shall call me from generation to generation."* (Exodus 3:14-15). God's glory is precious and jealously guarded. *"I am the Lord; that is my name! I will not yield my glory to another or my praise to idols."* (Isaiah 42:8). In no way is God's glory to be shared. There is none like Him.

The Psalmist proclaimed, *"Be exalted, O God, above the heavens; let your glory be over all the earth."* (Psalm 57:11). Jesus the Son of God *"is the radiance of God's glory and the exact representation of his being, sustaining all things by his powerful word."* (Hebrews 1:3).

God's glory is manifest in all creation. *"Yours, Lord, is the greatness and the power and the glory and the majesty and the splendor, for everything in heaven and earth is yours."* (1 Chronicles 29:11). The living creatures in heaven sing their praises *"You are worthy, our Lord and God, to receive glory and honor and power, for you created all things, and by your will they were created and have their being."* (Revelation 4:11).

The majesty of God's glory is reflected in His light. Isaiah proclaimed, *"Arise, shine, for your light has come, and the glory of the Lord rises upon you. ... The sun will no more be your light by day, nor will the brightness of the moon shine on you, for the Lord will be your everlasting light, and your God will be your glory."* (Isaiah 60:1,19).

Perhaps John Piper sums up best, "So God's glory is the radiance of his holiness, the radiance of his manifold, infinitely worthy and valuable perfections."[2]

Responding to God's Glory

The Shorter Catechism of the Westminster Confessions declares "Man's chief end is to glorify God, and to enjoy Him forever. ... The Word of God which is contained in the Scriptures of the Old and New Testaments is the only rule to direct us how we may glorify and enjoy Him."[3]

The Psalmists call upon us to *"Sing the glory* of his name; make his praise glorious."* (Psalm 66:2). *"I will praise God's name in song and glorify* him with thanksgiving."* (Psalm 69:30).

King David worshiped the Lord, *"Give praise to the Lord, proclaim his name; make known among the nations what he has done. Sing to him, sing praise to him; tell of all his wonderful acts."* (1 Chronicles 16:8-9).

Paul reminds us *"for all have sinned and fall short of the glory of God, and all are justified freely by his grace through the redemption that came by Christ Jesus."* (Romans 3:23-24). Therefore, we have every reason to glorify and praise God for we have received the gift of salvation by grace through Jesus Christ.

More than ever Paul encouraged us *"to live lives worthy of God."* (1 Thessalonians 2:12). *"So whether you eat or drink or whatever you do, do it all for the glory* of God."* (1 Corinthians 10:31). Jesus in the Sermon on the Mount instructs us *"In the same way, let your light shine before others, that they may see your good deeds and glorify* your Father in heaven."*

(Matthew 5:16). "To God be the Glory" in all that we do constitutes our act of worship, thanksgiving and praise for His name.

An application in healing

Billy Graham reminds us "Yet in the midst of trials we can thank God because we know He has promised to be with us, and He will help us. We know that he can use times of suffering to draw us closer to Himself."[4]

John Piper writing in *Don't Waste Your Cancer* drew attention to the hope of a new creation, and of His purpose in cancer. Christ has taken the curse of our diseases so that we may find comfort in Him. Even when we should think of death, we should cherish the moment to be with Christ. Cancer awakens us to the reality of God, to the opportunity to witness to the truth and glory of Christ.[5]

We give thanks to God for His grace in salvation and in healing. In all things God deserves our praise and worship. Soli Deo Gloria.

To him who is able to keep you from stumbling and to present you before his glorious presence without fault and with great joy — to the only God our Saviour be glory, majesty, power and authority, through Jesus Christ our Lord, before all ages, now and forevermore! Amen.
(Jude 1:24-25)

*****

REFERENCES

1. Boice, J. M. (2001). *Whatever Happened To The Gospel Of Grace.* Wheaton, Illinois, USA: Crossway Books. p 158
2. Piper, J. (2009, July 6). *What Is God's Glory?* Retrieved November 13, 2017 from Desiring God: https://www.desiringgod.org/interviews/what-is-gods-glory
3. The Westminster Confession of Faith, The Shorter Catechism. Q1, Q2

4. Graham, B. (1996). *Breakfast with Billy Graham.* Ann Arbor, Michigan, USA: Servant Publications. p 97

5. Piper, J. (2011). *Don't Waste Your Cancer.* Wheaton, Illinois, USA: Crossway. p 11

10
REFLECTIONS

There is a time for everything,
and a season for every activity under the heavens:
a time to be born and a time to die,
a time to plant and a time to uproot,
a time to kill and a time to heal,
ECCLESIASTES 3:1-3

I am now in a new season of my life. The active life in pursuit of work and recreation requires a change. There are to be changes in purpose, outlook and the things I do given the energy levels that I now have. There is the on-going concern and awareness of cancer and its possibility of return. For now I can savour the good news that I am free from cancer.

Many of my friends tell me that God has a purpose for me and that I am not done yet. To be useful is a nice and comforting thought. The question remains, for what?

My Limited Time Available

The great uncertainty is the time I have available to fulfil whatever I need to do in response to God's call. I do not know when the Lord will call me home. The general prognosis for pancreatic cancer is not particularly good. The reports I read of surviving pancreatic cancer do not suggest an extended life expectancy.

The American Cancer Society, based on data collected between 1992 and 1998, reported that the 5-year survival rate for Stage IIB cancer of this nature is about 5%. This means that in a population of 100, only five lived longer than five years after being diagnosed.[1]

I have had my operation to remove my tumours and have been declared cancer free. Under the circumstances, I could beat the odds and enjoy a longer life expectancy. These things however are in the hands of the Lord.

God's Creation and Purpose

As I reflect on my cancer and mull over whatever time remains for me, the Lord opened my eyes and brought me to realise how intricately and wonderfully made we all are. Each and every little organ within our bodies fulfils a specific function. The functions of every little organ are so specifically defined that they must have been divinely designed. There are no duplicates or spare parts within our bodies.

We have brains that absorb information, converting it into knowledge and interpreting knowledge to provide wisdom. Out of all of these we evoke feelings and emotions, reacting with others and memories that keep us grounded to life's realities. For some, we grow and live to our ripe old age.

Nothing within us is mechanical or robotic. Man may build machines and robots to help in doing work, but none of them can grow or work independently without human intervention. The field of Artificial Intelligence appears to enable machines to retain memory and knowledge of facts and events but beyond these functions the ability to draw on wisdom and emotions would be quite another matter altogether. Wisdom and emotions are what make us human and in the image of God.

Understanding God's Purpose

In the book of Genesis, the Bible tells us that God made man in His image (Genesis 1:26-27). We are made not just in physical form but we have also inherited some of His attributes – our ability to love and have compassion for others. We are not perfect, not because of God's design error, but because man, given a free will, chose to sin and rebel against God. Instead of life, sin brought us death and separation from God.

As I reflect on creation and Adam's fall through disobedience, I could not help but appreciate the need to be reconciled with a holy God. Had God not sent His Son Jesus, what would become of me when I die? I am a sinner and God is holy. What an unbridgeable gap there is in between.

My thoughts go out to those receiving chemotherapy with me at the Cancer Centre. What thoughts and fears run through their minds as they sat on those recliners? Do they fear death and the uncertainties thereafter? Do they know Jesus? Do they know that God loves them too? Like them my time is limited but I know the answers to those questions.

Whatever the time I have left, I am grateful to the Lord for this healing I received. I am mortal and so it would only be a matter of when, not if, that I should depart this world. I have the comfort and peace of knowing that I am saved by the grace of God.

Treasured Thoughts and Belongings

It is essential that I address what I consider important now. To me, God's work to which I am called is spending time with my family and strengthening of relationships therein. Equally important is time with friends and sharing the love of Jesus with those who do not yet know Him.

I have but only a few material treasures. These are mainly my books and collection of music in vinyl records. Many of these date back to the 1950s and 1960s, more than fifty or sixty years old. These are now collectors' items, no longer in production. Most of the artistes have also passed away. Many of the records were inherited from my father from a time when entertainment meant listening to music at home in the midst of noisy distractions elsewhere in the house or outside on the street. TV and sound proofed air-con rooms did not exist then. Yes, those were the good old days and I do miss them.

Being Called Home

The reality for cancer patients like myself must be to addess our end-of-life issues. Preparations for our final moments are practical issues best put to rest when we are still alive, conscious and able to express our thoughts and desires.

Perhaps a most sensitive matter to be dealt with in the event of physical death and separation from family has to do with funeral arrangements and what to do with my remains. After cremation I wish for my ashes are to be scattered in the sea. There is a practical reason for this.

I have over the years, in land scarce Singapore, experienced countless exhumations and transfers of the remains of my loved ones who have passed away. Not counting the emotional toll, the costs and inconvenience involved are significant.

I am of the mindset that those who will remember me would likely extend only to my grandson's generation. Even then, memories will be fleeting and fade with time. King Solomon acknowledges *"No one remembers the former generations, and even those yet to come will not be remembered by those who follow them."* (Ecclesiastes **1:11**)

These are the hard truths of life. The future generations have their lives to live and challenges to contend with. A grave or even a columbarium niche in Singapore would be too much to manage. Under the circumstances, it is best that no physical memorial is retained to house my remains.

God's Sovereignty and Grace

This leads me back to some contemplative thoughts: What then is the meaning of life? Why am I cleared of cancer and why am I healed? What is it with the extension of my life?

My doctors can offer only a medical explanation. The treatment I received worked. I am thankful for their skills and their efforts. I would certainly be in a worse state without God's miracles in advanced medical science.

I am grateful for all my family and friends and especially, my prayer warriors who encouraged me and gave me emotional and spiritual support. Without them it would have been a lonely battle with possibilities of depression and loss of hope.

These events I come to acknowledge explain more how I have been healed but does not answer the question "why". I have seen and know of friends and loved ones who did not survive cancer. Some went into remission only to see the return of cancer taking over their lives.

It is probably too early for me to claim success and victory in my battle with cancer. I do not have an answer for whatever the reason that God has healed me, in this season. From my spiritual perspective, He has healed me for His purpose and for His glory. By His grace, I have been healed.

Why have I been healed and not others? The answers to these questions are known only to God. I shall not speculate. The evidence over the past year since I was first diagnosed points to His constant presence and interventions in my healing process. His grace is made more precious and tangible through my cancer.

As I reflect on and relate this story, I can only say for sure that God's grace was there for me. His love and compassion were displayed through all who were involved in my treatment and recovery. Everything was in God's time and in His will for me. It was God's favour upon me. He has given me a new reason and a new season for living.

One purpose I know that has been on my mind and in my heart as I progress through my treatment is to relate this journey, to declare His love for me and for each of us. He has revealed His wonderful grace in the midst of my cancer. More than ever it is my desire to glorify Him and praise Him for being the gracious and compassionate God to me.

I am here but only for a season. There is a time for everything. When my purpose is done, and the Lord calls me home, my season comes to an end. My work here would have been done. I may be separated from my loved ones here on earth but the Lord would have a much better place for me. For us who believe in Jesus, we shall all one day share in His glory and be reunited again.

We shall all meet again as the beautiful hymn, *In the Sweet By and By*, proclaims:

There's a land that is fairer than day,
And by faith we can see it afar;
For the Father waits over the way
To prepare us a dwelling place there.

Refrain:
In the sweet by and by,
We shall meet on that beautiful shore;
In the sweet by and by,
We shall meet on that beautiful shore[2]

*****

REFERENCES

1. American Cancer Society. (2017). Pancreatic Cancer Survival Rates, By Stage. Retrieved July 12, 2017 from American Cancer Society: https://www.cancer.org/cancer/pancreatic-cancer/detection-diagnosis-staging/survival-rates.html
2. Bennett, S. F. (1868). In The Sweet By and By. (Public Domain) Retrieved July 13, 2017 from Timeless Truths: http://library.timelesstruths.org/music/In_the_Sweet_By_and_By/

*****

EPILOGUE

As I close the writing of this book, it is December 2017. My cancer has returned.

At the end of August 2017, my blood test results revealed an elevated cancer marker. My oncologist was concerned and ordered a review in October. This time the cancer markers have advanced significantly. My CT scan showed the spread of cancer to my liver. Based on staging conventions, I am now into Stage IV pancreatic cancer. The prognosis was not promising.

There were several options to treating the cancer. These include immunotherapy, chemotherapy and in some cases, patients look to alternative medicine and treatment.

Treatment under immunotherapy involves participation in clinical trials. On learning more about the treatment, my family and I grew less comfortable about being part of the process. We prayed. As it turned out, my biopsy results indicated that my cancer was not suitable for the drugs involved. The Lord has seemingly closed that door.

I am now scheduled to start oral chemotherapy on the third week of December just before Christmas.

Pancreatic cancer is particularly aggressive and known to recur. Did the Lord heal me of cancer?

My personal view is that the Lord intervened to give me half a year of being free from cancer. I was not on any cancer treatment and was able to lead a normal life. This condition applies to only less than ten per cent of patients in my condition. I am thankful for the time given to me.

The return of my cancer was a sombre disappointment. We have no explanation why it resurfaced. I was briefly discouraged and depressed. However, I realised that God is in control and whatever the outcome and results, I can rest in His sovereignty and grace. We continue to pray in the hope of His healing hands to be upon me and for wisdom and guidance.

I give thanks to the Lord for giving me all these years and even for this extra year and more following my initial diagnosis. My pancreatic cancer could have been a silent killer growing within me without my knowledge had it not been exposed. I now have every opportunity to fight it and to secure victory over it by His grace. My Lord is my shield and my strength. *"The Lord will fight for you; you need only to be still."* (Exodus 14:14)

Whatever the outcome, we place our trust in the Lord for His will to be done and for His purpose in me to be fulfilled. Amen.

*I press on toward the goal to win the prize for which God
has called me heavenward in Christ Jesus.* (Phil 3:14)

*****

ABOUT THE AUTHOR

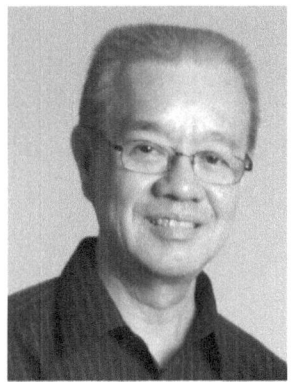

Michael Swee-Lim Seah

A child of God, a sinner saved by grace.

Michael, 71, is a member of Adam Road Presbyterian Church, Singapore. He serves in the Brothers and Sisters Keepers (BASK) ministry under the Mercy Ministry of the church.

In 2004 Michael joined Bible Study Fellowship and shortly thereafter was called to be a Children Leader in the BSF School Programme. He stepped down at the end of 2017 following treatment for cancer

www.ingramcontent.com/pod-product-compliance
Lightning Source LLC
Chambersburg PA
CBHW050356290526
45786CB00003B/1016